SEX, SIN, AND SCIENCE

Recent Titles in
Healing Society: Disease, Medicine, and History
John Parascandola, Series Editor

From Snake Oil to Medicine: Pioneering Public Health
R. Alton Lee

A History of Multiple Sclerosis
Colin Talley

SEX, SIN, AND SCIENCE

A HISTORY OF SYPHILIS IN AMERICA

JOHN PARASCANDOLA

Foreword by Richard H. Carmona

Healing Society: Disease, Medicine, and History
John Parascandola, Series Editor

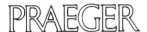

Westport, Connecticut
London

Library of Congress Cataloging-in-Publication Data

Parascandola, John, 1941–
   Sex, sin, and science : a history of syphilis in America / John Parascandola.
     p. ; cm. — (Healing society—disease, medicine, and history, ISSN 1933-5938)
   Includes bibliographical references and index.
   ISBN-13: 978–0–275–99430–3 (alk. paper)
   1. Syphilis—United States—History.
   [DNLM: 1. Syphilis—history—United States.   WC 160 P223s 2008]   I. Title.
   II. Series.
   RC201.5.A2P37   2008
   616.95'13—dc22   2008009953

British Library Cataloguing in Publication Data is available.

Library of Congress Catalog Card Number: 2008009953
ISBN-13: 978–0–275–99430–3
ISSN: 1933-5938

First published in 2008

Praeger Publishers, 88 Post Road West, Westport, CT 06881
An imprint of Greenwood Publishing Group, Inc.
www.praeger.com

Printed in the United States of America

The paper used in this book complies with the
Permanent Paper Standard issued by the National
Information Standards Organization (Z39.48–1984).

10 9 8 7 6 5 4 3 2 1

For my wife Randee

CONTENTS

FOREWORD

HISTORY OF SYPHILIS IN AMERICA

Dr. John Parascandola, former Public Health Service Historian and an accomplished scholar and author, once again has produced a thoughtful, powerful, and revealing treatise, this time on the history of syphilis in the "new world." However, the title may be misleading in that this text on syphilis covers more than the history of the disease itself, but also provides the viewer a unique vantage point into the social, economic, political, and value systems of our evolving nation over several centuries. Addressing the science of syphilis alone would create a book devoid of this nation's tumultuous history as well as dissecting the spirochete nakedly out of context. For we know that the public health history of any disease, especially sexually transmitted diseases, is inextricably intertwined with the era of occurrence and the prevalent culture of that time.

The history of syphilis and its pathogen, *Treponema pallidum*, is fascinating and its origin is still debated in various theories, with questions raised about whether or not it originated in the new world and then traveled to Europe in the fifteenth century via explorers returning home. Syphilis has plagued communities and nations as well as undermined national defense as it did in 1495 when the French troops were infected as they attacked Naples, and as it threatened our own troops, especially during World Wars I and II as well as in Korea and Vietnam.

Many well-known global figures over the centuries have had syphilis. This would include but not be limited to King Henry the VIII, Howard Hughes, Al Capone, Paul Gaugin, Vladimir Lenin, and many, many more.

Syphilis has also been described as the "great imitator" since in its primary, secondary, and tertiary forms it can mimic many diseases. Both before and after the germ theory was promulgated, syphilis has always caused very divisive and charged debates even through today. Through the ages it has usually been the social and cultural and not the scientific context of syphilis that has hampered the health of populations in the United States and globally, as well as threatened the careers of many public health officers, including Surgeons General. For the public health science of any disease may often conflict with the theological, ideological, or political environment of any given era.

This has certainly been demonstrated by syphilis over the ages, as exemplified by the disease being attributed to dirty immigrants, immoral persons, or racial groups (e.g., blacks with supposedly inferior health being characterized as "a syphilis soaked race"). Other illogical but very potent ideologies of the time have also had a chilling effect on those who would speak out against the nonscientific bias. Dr. Parascandola masterfully steers us through this complete maze of evolving global social norms and history and science over centuries so that the challenge of syphilis is presented in context.

It has been said that history is a prologue to our future. In syphilis we see the truth in the statement as well as its application to many other contemporary health challenges such as AIDS.

There is a much bigger picture here than syphilis alone that the general public, historians, politicians, and science can benefit from.

Hopefully, an enlightened society can recognize the errors of the past in order to create the future we so desperately need.

Richard H. Carmona, M.D., M.P.H., FACS
17th Surgeon General of the United States (2002–2006)

SERIES FOREWORD

The Praeger series *Healing Society: Disease, Medicine, and History* features individual volumes that explore the social impact of particular illnesses or medically related conditions or topics for a broad audience. The object is to publish books that offer reliable overviews of particular aspects of medical and social history while incorporating the most up-to-date scholarly interpretations. The books in the series are designed to engage readers and educate them about important but often neglected aspects of the social history of medicine. Disease and disability have significantly influenced the course of human history, and the books in this series will examine various aspects of that influence.

Diseases, and how we react to them, are shaped by social and cultural factors as well as medical ones, and the history of syphilis, because of the association of the disease with sex and all of the moral views surrounding sex, particularly reflects this theme. The present book traces the history of syphilis in the United States from colonial times to the present. Several themes explored in the book illustrate ways in which nonmedical factors influence our views of a disease and our reaction to it. One of these themes is the tendency to focus blame for the spread of a disease on a particular group (e.g., women, blacks, sinners). The balance between protecting the rights of individuals and protecting the public health, in issues such as whether to quarantine the infected and whether to require mandatory testing for the disease, is another theme. A third theme is the persistent reluctance of many Americans to discuss venereal disease openly because it involves sex, a subject that we are generally fascinated with but often not comfortable talking about. The story of syphilis in America is a fascinating tale of tension between sex, sin, and science.

ACKNOWLEDGMENTS

The research for this book was conducted at a number of libraries and archives, and I am grateful to the staffs of the following institutions for their assistance: Social Welfare History Archives, Elmer L. Andersen Library, University of Minnesota, Minneapolis, MN (especially David Klaassen); National Archives and Records Administration, Southeast Region, Morrow, GA (especially Maryann Hawkins, Richard Rayburn, and Robert Richards); National Archives and Records Administration, College Park, MD (especially Marjorie Ciarlante and Tab Lewis); Archives Service Center, University of Pittsburgh, Pittsburgh, PA (especially Marianne Kasica, as well as Jonathon Erlen of the University of Pittsburgh for assisting me in accessing the Thomas Parran Papers); National Library of Medicine, Bethesda, MD.

Many colleagues provided me with useful references, suggestions, and other helpful advice over the years that I was carrying out the research for this book, for which I am grateful, but they are too numerous to list here, and I would no doubt inadvertently leave someone out if I tried. I appreciate the assistance of Brian Foster of Praeger in getting the book through production. Finally, I wish to thank Elizabeth Demers (formerly of Praeger) and my wife Randee for reading the entire manuscript, calling my attention to errors, and making suggestions for improvement.

INTRODUCTION

Syphilis is the killer-not swiftly, but after long years of pain and invalidism, often insanity. It has been known to doctors since the time of Columbus, whose ships, some historians believe, brought the plague back to Europe where it raged as the "Great Pox" in the wake of wars almost as devastating as those of today. The germ which causes it is called the spirochete. Under the microscope it looks like a tiny wriggling corkscrew.[1]

VD [venereal disease] as the theme of a book ought to have all the terror and fascination of murder and bubonic plague and more, because it is inescapably tied to sex. Sex is now and perhaps has always been the most engrossing of all subjects.[2]

We understand diseases not only as medical entities. Social, cultural, and economic forces also "frame" the ways in which we view diseases.[3] An individual disease may be perceived in different ways in different societies and time periods, with both scientific and cultural factors affecting our view of the disease and our reaction to it. The association of "dirt" with disease, for example, has long shaped our perception of various illnesses. Poliomyelitis (polio) was associated with filth and flies well into the twentieth century, even after the discovery of the virus responsible for the disease. The public often looks for groups to blame for diseases, especially when epidemics strike, and in the case of polio, immigrants were the scapegoat. In the late nineteenth and early decades of the twentieth century, when many Americans were concerned about the large-scale immigration of people from southern and eastern Europe, health officials blamed the spread of polio on the unsanitary and even immoral habits of these immigrants. This theory of the transmission of the disease fit the antiimmigrant, nativist mood of the country. Nor have such sentiments completely disappeared from our society. Naomi Rogers has written:

> The fear of dirt and its association with disease persists into our own world.... The long-held connection between dirt and disease did not just disappear with widespread knowledge of the germ theory. It continues to hold a powerful intellectual and practical appeal: it combines morality and science; it helps to distinguish rich from poor, native-born from immigrant, the ignorant and careless from the informed and responsible.[4]

Consumption (as tuberculosis was formerly known) was long attributed to a constitutional weakness and unhealthy habits or surroundings. With the development of the germ theory of disease and the isolation of the tubercle bacillus (1882), tuberculosis became a communicable disease that was caused by a specific microorganism. Although this new understanding of the disease led to some difference in attitudes toward patients and in treatment, other factors still affected how tuberculosis was viewed. In the early part of the twentieth century, for example, medical authorities still tended to ascribe the high mortality rates of African Americans from tuberculosis to "racial characteristics," reflecting a general bias that blacks had inferior constitutions and health.[5]

Whether or not a particular condition or behavior is defined as a disease can change over time. Alcoholism, for example, went from being considered a bad habit to being classified as a disease, although not without controversy. In the nineteenth century, masturbation was considered to be a disease. By the end of that century, the medical profession had come to view homosexuality as a disease. This view remained official psychiatric doctrine into the 1970s. Concepts of sexual morality obviously helped to shape some of these classifications.[6]

Social and cultural factors also influence the way in which we react to a disease and to those who suffer from it, as already suggested above. Leprosy (or Hansen's Disease) is a particularly striking example of such a case. It is disease that is almost noncontagious, generally requiring prolonged and intimate contact with an infected person for the disease to be communicated to another person. Yet the disease acquired a stigma, perhaps because it could be disfiguring and was considered "unclean," that led to an irrational fear of persons with this condition, a fear that continued long after medical science showed that the disease was rarely transmitted from one person to another. People with leprosy were shunned and often forced to live in confinement. Even today the disease is often used as a metaphor for disgrace or disgust, as when one man with AIDS said that he "was feeling ashamed and like a leper" or when an athlete indicted in the steroid scandal was described as a "baseball leper."[7]

In the case of a disease associated with sex, social and cultural factors unsurprisingly figure large in its history. Religious and moral views, for example, influence essentially everything connected with sex, and that includes sexually transmitted diseases. The term "sexually transmitted diseases" is a relatively recent one. Historically these maladies have been known as venereal diseases, the term that will generally be used in this book. "Venereal" ultimately derives from the Latin name of the goddess of love, Venus.

Until the advent of AIDS in the 1980s, by far the most serious of the venereal diseases was syphilis. The purpose of this book is to examine the fascinating history of this disease in the United States, placing it within a broader social context. Although I believe the work will be of interest to professional historians interested in medicine and public health, my goal has been to write a book that will be accessible and appealing to a broad general audience. I have not assumed any specialized knowledge of the history of medicine on the past of the reader, and have tried to provide the background necessary for understanding the story of this disease. The book is based on extensive research in both the primary and secondary literature. The most original contributions to scholarship are in the chapters dealing with the history of syphilis in twentieth-century America, which draw substantially on primary sources.

Although the book is concerned primarily with the history of syphilis in America, I thought it necessary to include background information on the origins of the disease and its spread in Europe. The first chapter therefore introduces the disease and discusses its history in Europe from the time that it made its first appearance at the end of the fifteenth century to the beginning of the twentieth century.

The succeeding chapters trace the history of syphilis in America in chronological order. Chapter 2 covers the period from colonial times up to World War I. Chapters 3, 4, and 5 discuss syphilis in World War I, the interwar years, and World War II, respectively. The final chapter deals with the post-World War II era, bringing the story up to the present day. Although the focus throughout is on syphilis, it will frequently be considered in the broader context of venereal disease in general since many social policies, public concerns, preventive methods, etc. applied to other sexually transmitted diseases as well.

There are a number of themes explored in the book that illustrate ways in which social and cultural factors affect our view of disease and our reaction to it. One of these themes is the tendency to focus blame for the spread of the disease on a particular group. Over the centuries, for example, women (especially prostitutes and so-called promiscuous women) were traditionally singled out as being primarily responsible for the transmission of syphilis and other venereal diseases. African Americans were viewed by many whites as being a "syphilis-soaked" race. Blaming the victims, whatever their gender or race, for acquiring the disease because of their own sinful behavior has also been a thread in the history of venereal disease. All of these practices reflect particular stereotypes and moral views.

The balance between protecting the rights of individuals and protecting the public health, in issues such as whether to quarantine the infected and whether to require

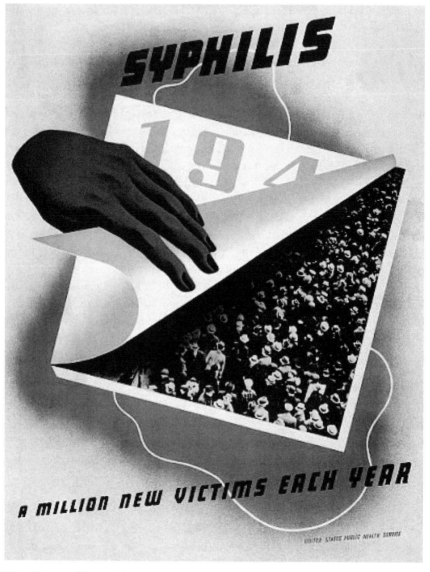

United States Public Health Service syphilis poster, 1941 [Courtesy of the National Library of Medicine].

mandatory testing for the disease, is another theme. This conflict, like the tendency to blame a particular segment of society for spreading a disease, is not unique to venereal diseases, but pervades much of public health practice. It is a dilemma that we still confront today, as witnessed by the recent action by the government of South Africa to forcibly confine patients infected with especially lethal strains of tuberculosis in prison-like hospitals.[8] The story of syphilis, however, provides some compelling examples of this tension between civil liberties and state police powers. In times of war, as the history of venereal disease demonstrates, the pendulum tends to shift more in the direction of the state over the individual.

A third theme is the persistent reluctance of many Americans to discuss venereal disease openly because it involves sex, a subject that we are often not comfortable talking about in spite of living in a culture that at times seems to be obsessed with all things sexual. Moral and religious views of sex have shaped the attitudes of many toward syphilis and other venereal diseases. The use of condoms to protect against sexually transmitted diseases, for example, is opposed by those who are against birth control or who fear that this use will encourage promiscuity. Throughout America's history, there have been those who criticized any explicit education about sex and venereal disease because nice people do not talk about such things, or because teenagers should not be exposed to materials on sex, or for various other reasons.

I hope that the reader of this book will come away with not just a better understanding of the history of syphilis, but also with an appreciation for the complex ways in which societies categorize diseases and those who suffer from them, as well as a sense of how our reaction to diseases is shaped by our broader social and cultural values. I would like to think that I have also told a good story that makes for enjoyable reading.

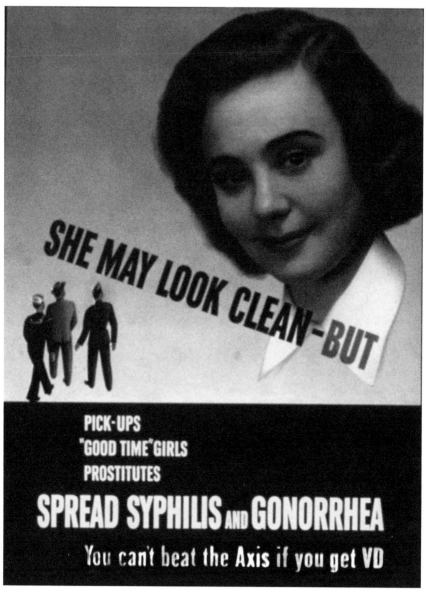

World War II American poster warning servicemen that you could not tell whether or not a woman had a venereal disease by her appearance. Women traditionally have been assigned an unfair share of the blame for spreading venereal disease [Courtesy of the National Library of Medicine].

ONE

THE GREAT POX: ORIGINS AND EUROPEAN BACKGROUND

ORIGINS OF THE DISEASE

Shortly after Columbus had arrived in the New World, as the fifteenth century drew to a close, a terrible new disease appeared in Europe. One early medical commentator described the malady in the following graphic terms:

> The signs of the sickness are these: there are itching sensations and an unpleasant pain in the joints; there is a rapidly increasing fever; the skin is inflamed with revolting scabs, and is completely covered with swellings and tubercules which are initially of a livid red color, and then become blacker. After a few days a sanguine humor oozes out; this is followed by excrescences which look like tiny sponges which have been squeezed dry. . . . It most often begins with the private parts.[1]

This previously unknown disease, which frequently began in the "private parts" of the victim, made its first significant appearance in Naples in 1495, near the beginning of a series of "Italian Wars" that engulfed Europe for about a half-century. The conflict began in 1494, when Ludovico Sforza seized the throne of the Duchy of Milan. He was opposed by the ruler of the Kingdom of Naples, who also had a claim on the Duchy. Sforza decided to ally himself with Charles VIII, the King of France, in an effort to remove the threat from Naples. He encouraged Charles, who had a claim to Naples, to invade Italy and march on Naples when its ruler died in 1494. Charles' army, consisting largely of mercenaries, advanced quickly through Italy with little opposition and captured Naples in February of 1495.

Charles' sack of Naples finally provoked a reaction against the French. Even Sforza now feared that Charles, who could also lay claim to Milan, might decide to annex other Italian city-states in addition to Naples. The Pope put together the League of Venice, which included Spain and the Holy Roman Empire in addition to Milan and Venice, to drive the French out of Italy. Charles did not want to be trapped in Naples, so he marched his army north to Lombardy, where he engaged the forces of the League of Venice at the Battle of Fornovo on July 5, 1495. The battle did not go well for the French and Charles retreated to his own country.[2]

When the mercenary soldiers of Charles' army disbanded and returned to their respective countries, they carried with them the new disease. In fact, Charles himself fell victim to this malady. An early description of the disease was provided by doctors to the Venetian troops at Fornovo, who wrote of "pustules" on the faces and bodies of some of the soldiers, followed by intense pain in various parts of the body. Less than a decade after this battle, the disease had spread throughout Europe. Early descriptions of the symptoms of the disease generally mention the presence of pustules, boils, and ulcers on the body and pain, sometimes intense, in the joints. In the worst cases, the sores could "eat away" the nose or other parts of the face and body.[3]

Understandably, no one was anxious to claim "credit" for this scourge. Because many believed that the disease first made it appearance in the French troops besieging Naples, it was often called (especially by the Italians) *morbus gallicus* ("French disease"), and this was perhaps the most common designation in the early history of the disease. The French, on the other hand, preferred to call it the "Neapolitan disease," blaming it on the city of Naples. It soon came to be called by other names as well, including the "bubas" (after the sores produced by the disease), the "pox" or the "great pox" (to distinguish it from smallpox).[4]

This disease has come to be identified as syphilis. The understanding and categorization of disease in the fifteenth and sixteenth centuries was far different than it is today, and some have pointed out that references to epidemics of the French disease in this period might have included other diseases along with syphilis. In addition, the disease syphilis has undoubtedly changed over the centuries, a not infrequent occurrence with respect to diseases caused by microorganisms that can mutate over time. The descriptions of the symptoms of the great pox and its mortality in this early period indicate a disease that manifested itself more severely than syphilis today. For our purposes, however, we shall accept the traditional interpretation of the pox as syphilis.[5]

Although there were some scholars who attempted to identify this malady with disease descriptions in the ancient literature, the majority of the early commentators agreed that the pox was indeed a new disease, never before seen in Europe. But how did this disease come into being, and why had it afflicted Europe at this time? One

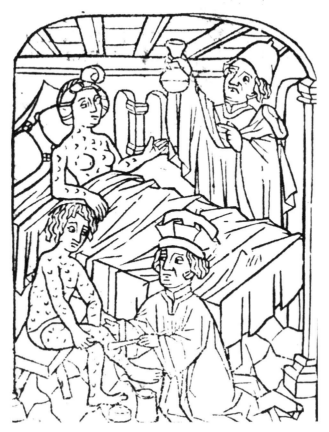

Physicians examining and treating patients with syphilis. From Bartholomäus Steber, *A malafranczos morbo Gallorum praeservatio ac cura* (Vienna, 1497–98) [Courtesy of the National Library of Medicine].

of the initial reactions to this malady was that it was a punishment from God. The Holy Roman Emperor Maximilian issued an edict already in 1495 stating that the "evil pocks" had not been seen before and had been sent by God as a punishment for blasphemy.[6] In the fifteenth century, it was commonly believed that diseases were often a result of God's displeasure. The court physician of Ferrara, Italy, for example, wrote in 1497 in reference to the French disease, "We also see that the Supreme Creator, now full of wrath against us for our dreadful sins, punishes us with this cruelest of ills, which has now spread not only through Italy but across the whole of Christendom."[7] The noted sixteenth-century French surgeon Ambroise Paré also believed that the disease was a sign of God's wrath at the sins of mankind.[8]

Other explanations were also offered for the advent of this plague. An Italian chronicler who was secretary to several popes believed that the French disease had been transmitted by the Jews, many of whom had settled in Naples after being expelled from Spain in 1492. He compared the situation to the introduction of leprosy by the Jews, in his view, when they were driven out of Egypt. Jews had also served as scapegoats during the Black Death (bubonic plague) epidemics of the fourteenth century, when they were accused of poisoning the wells to cause the disease. In the late eighteenth century, Christian Gottfried Gruner built upon the Jewish theory to suggest that syphilis first appeared among the *Marrani*, a term he used to include both the Jews and the Arabs who were expelled from Spain in 1492.[9]

A particularly popular explanation for the disease was that it was caused by astrological factors. Astrology was accepted not only by laymen at the time, but many doctors also made use of astrology in their practice. Not surprisingly then, astrology was called upon to help understand the origins of this new and devastating disease. Especially influential in this regard were the 1495 treatises on pox by the German physician Joseph Grünpeck. Admitting that God's will was the first cause of the pox, Grünpeck saw astrology as the second or physical case of the disease. He traced the advent of the French disease to a conjunction of the planets Saturn and Jupiter on November 25, 1484 that portended disastrous developments. Although this event had occurred some ten years before the beginning of the syphilis epidemic, Grünpeck relied on other properties of the planets to manipulate his data and provide an astrological explanation for the disease.[10]

COLUMBIAN CONNECTION

Although syphilis first appeared in Europe soon after Columbus had returned to Spain from his first voyage to America, it does not appear that anyone, at least in print, attempted to connect the two events until 1526. In that year, the Spanish nobleman Gonzalo Fernandez de Oviedo y Valdes, who was at the royal court when Ferdinand and Isabella greeted Columbus upon his return, published his *Natural History of the Indies*. This work was based upon Oviedo's experiences in the Americas as superintendent of the Spanish silver and gold mines and as governor of the castle of Santo Domingo.[11] In a statement in the book addressed to the King of Spain, Oviedo wrote:

> Your majesty may take it as certain that this malady (the bubas) comes from the Indes, where it is very common among the Indians, but not so dangerous in those lands as it is in our own. . . . The first time this sickness was seen in Spain was after Admiral Don Christopher Columbus had discovered the Indes and returned from those lands. Some Christians among those who went with him and took part in the discovery, and the many more who made the second trip, brought back this scourge, and from them it was passed on to others.[12]

In 1539, another Spaniard, physician Diaz de Isla, provided further support for this view in a book on the pox, arguing that the disease first appeared in Europe in Barcelona after the return of Columbus. He claimed that he had treated sailors from Columbus' voyage and others with the disease in Barcelona.[13] Blaming foreigners for a disease has been a common practice throughout history. We have already seen how the Italians called syphilis the French disease, while the French called it the Neapolitan disease. The Japanese blamed the Chinese, the Russians the Poles, and the Persians the Turks for the spread of the pox. Placing the blame on American Indians removed the stigma from Europe entirely, assigning responsibility to an external "Other" (the Indian).[14]

The theory that syphilis originated in America ignited a dispute that has lasted some 500 years, as the matter has still not been completely resolved. The debate, which began in earnest in the seventeenth century, tilted heavily in favor of those who supported the American origin in the eighteenth century. In his 1736 book on syphilis, French royal physician Jean Astruc made a strong case for the disease having originated on the West Indian island of Santo Domingo, where the crew of Columbus supposedly came into contact with it. Cultural factors undoubtedly helped win the day for the American theory, as three historians have pointed out in a recent book.

> The rise of European consciousness in the eighteenth century convinced Europeans that the pox had come from outside Europe and had arisen there among outsiders. This made the theory of a New World origin of the pox attractive; it also made it possible to believe that it originated among others seen as outsiders, like the Jews and Arabs who had been expelled from Spain at the end of the fifteenth century.[15]

From then on, historian of syphilis Jacques Quétel contends, the theory of the American origin of the disease was firmly established and supported by the most eminent writers. However, opponents of this view continued to press their case.[16] It is beyond the scope of this book to trace this controversy in detail. Since information from the historical literature was unable to settle the question, hopes for resolving the dispute began to focus on looking for syphilitic lesions in bones and teeth once the scientific techniques for such research emerged in the last part of the nineteenth century. Over the course of the twentieth century, numerous skeletal remains were examined in the search for evidence of syphilis in the pre-Columbian period in America, Europe, and other parts of the world. The scale tipped back and forth with respect to the American origins theory as new discoveries were made and challenged. Although the methods for dating human remains have improved over time, thus narrowing the scope for disagreement over their age, the matter or whether or not a lesion is syphilitic is still open to interpretation. The study is complicated by the fact that other diseases, such as yaws and pinta, are caused by bacteria of the treponeme class to which the syphilis organism belongs, and can produce lesions similar to those of syphilis.

In recent years, the evidence seemed to be turning in favor of the view that syphilis was not brought to Europe from America, but existed in the Old World in some form before 1492. Newer molecular methods, based on DNA analysis, are allowing for a more positive identification of the syphilis organism. One article reviewing the recent literature on the controversy concluded that "Old World specimens with pathological alterations attributed to venereal syphilis and dated to pre-Columbian times seem to invalidate the Columbian theory and call for a more differentiated analysis of the phenomenon of syphilis than a theory based on a single factor can provide."[17] In a comprehensive multiauthored work on the history of treponeme diseases in North America before 1492, published in 2005 as *The Myth of Syphilis*, the editors conclude that although there is ample evidence from skeletal lesions that diseases caused by treponemes existed in the New World before Columbus arrived, there is no solid support for the view that a distinctly venereal type of syphilis was present in North America at that time. [18] In other words, they found no evidence for "the old theory that venereal syphilis was the New World's revenge upon Columbus and his crew."[19]

However, just as this book was going to press, molecular geneticists at Emory University reported that they had found evidence that supported the Columbian hypothesis. The Emory investigators, led by Kristin Harper, sequenced the DNA of a number of different strains of human *Treponema pallidum* (the bacterium that causes syphilis and related diseases such as yaws). They concluded that New World yaws belonged to a group distinct from Old World strains, and that based on genetic evidence it appeared likely that the New World strain was the intermediate between yaws and syphilis. The similarity between New World yaws and syphilis was especially evident in a variation of the yaws pathogen isolated recently from two children in a remote region of Guyana in South America. Harper claimed that these findings supported the idea that syphilis, or at least a progenitor of syphilis, originated in the Americas. Critics, however, have pointed out what they consider to be shortcomings in the methods and interpretations of the study, arguing, for example, that firm conclusions should not be based on two samples from one location in Guyana. It thus remains to be seen whether future research will settle once and for all this centuries-old debate.[20]

If the disease did not first enter Europe through contact with the Americas, the question remains as to why it seems to have made its first appearance in the Old World in the 1490s. It is possible that the *Treponema pallidum* organism, which undoubtedly was present in Europe before 1492, underwent a mutation at around that time to produce the apparently new disease of venereal syphilis. If syphilis did exist earlier in Europe, but not in epidemic proportions, perhaps it was generally misdiagnosed, confused with other diseases such as leprosy. Syphilis in fact came to be known as the "great imitator" because it often mimicked the symptoms of other diseases. But then why should the disease suddenly have become epidemic and been recognized as a new entity at the end of the fifteenth century? Some of the factors that have been suggested to explain the sudden spread of syphilis in this period include the movements of peoples across countries due to wars and voyages of exploration, hygienic conditions in areas that were urbanizing, and increasing sexual liberty. The invention of the Gutenberg printing press also meant that knowledge about the disease could be more rapidly diffused.[21]

SEX AND WOMEN

From soon after the first appearance of the French disease, many commentators began to associate its spread with sexual activity. As early as 1497, there were medical writers warning men against having sex with women who were infected with syphilis lest they themselves contract the disease. It must be remembered that the existence of microorganisms was unknown at this time, so of course the role of germs in disease was not understood. Disease was thought of, as it had been since antiquity, in terms of an imbalance of the four "humors" that make up the body (blood, phlegm, yellow bile, black bile). The equilibrium of these humors could be disturbed by a variety of factors, including diet and climate, causing a person to fall ill. Yet physicians did recognize that some diseases were contagious, i.e., could be passed on from one person to another, even though they did not understand the mechanism involved. People were therefore admonished to avoid contact with individuals who had the disease.[22]

Some doctors denied that one could be infected through sexual intercourse, even though the sores associated with syphilis frequently occurred first on the genitals. Evidence for the sexual transmission of syphilis began to mount, however, so that in the sixteenth century this view became generally accepted, although the idea that the disease could in addition be transmitted in other ways (e.g., by contact with the clothing or other effects of an infected person) was not ruled out. Although it was not clear how the disease spread, it was widely assumed to involve the introduction of some kind of poison into the body.[23]

The first person to have used the term *morbus venerus* ("venereal sickness") to refer to syphilis appears to have been the French physician Jacques de Béthencourt in 1527. He suggested this name because he thought that the disease should be named after its cause, which he believed to be the passions arising from immoral sex. The association of syphilis with sinful sexual activity was not uncommon from the early days of recognition of the disease on, and has not completely disappeared even today.[24] Syphilis was seen by some as a just reward for unbridled lust.[25] As Jacques Quétel noted in his history of syphilis, for many in the seventeenth century, "the pox and lechery go hand-in-hand."[26]

The association of syphilis with sex was not gender neutral, since women received the major portion of the blame for the disease and its spread. As early as 1497, the Italian physician Gaspar Torrella argued that men suffered more from the pox than did women because they have a hotter complexion. In addition, the uterus encouraged the corruption of vapors in infected women, and hence the spread of the disease. Men should therefore avoid having sex with infected women. However, according to Torrella, if an infected man had sexual relations with a woman who was infection-free, she was not likely to contract the disease because the cold, dry, and dense nature of the uterus meant that it did not suffer damage easily. Women would only become infected after repeated sexual contact with infected men.[27]

Historian Mary Spongberg has pointed out that after syphilis appeared women (especially promiscuous women) were generally regarded as the source of the disease in the popular mind, and that most medical authorities did not seem to be opposed to this view. It was believed by many that women could be exempt from the disease and yet pass it on to men, and that the symptoms of the disease were often hidden in women who did suffer from syphilis. Spongberg added, "The idea that men acquired venereal disease from women is taken for granted throughout the medical literature on the subject. Men are consistently represented as the victim of disease, women as its source."[28]

Such a view was consistent with a long tradition in Western thought, where women were associated with disease in general. The female body was seen as inferior to the male body going back to ancient Greece, and women were therefore viewed as being somehow abnormal and inherently diseased. The female genetalia were believed to be a lesser form of the male genetalia. Menstruation was generally represented as somehow morbid and polluting, and one early theory of syphilis associated the disease with a poison in menstrual blood.[29]

Prostitutes and promiscuous women were especially targeted as sources of syphilis. Already in 1497, even before the venereal nature of syphilis was firmly established in the medical community, the town Council of Aberdeen, Scotland, in an effort to combat the disease, ordered all "loose women" to desist from "the sins of venery" or they would be branded with a hot iron and banished from the town.[30] The practice of placing a major share of the blame for the spread of venereal disease on women, especially those whose morals were considered suspect, continued right up through the twentieth century.

The prostitute even came to be associated with the origins of syphilis in some popular lore. The controversial and colorful Swiss physician Paracelsus claimed in the 1530s that syphilis had originated as the result of sexual intercourse between a Frenchman with leprosy and a prostitute with uterine sores. Syphilis was not uncommonly associated with leprosy during this early period. Then in 1556 the Italian Pietro Rostino published a popular treatise on the pox in which he put forward a related theory on the origins of the disease. Rostino's account told of a beautiful prostitute who provided sexual services to the French troops that had invaded Italy in 1494. This prostitute had a putrefying sore at the opening of her womb. The rubbing of the penis of a male soldier against the sore caused the penis to break out in ulcers. In this manner, soldier after soldier was infected through intercourse with the prostitute, and the epidemic of syphilis had begun.[31]

There were of course moral reasons for the opposition to prostitution, but the spread of syphilis contributed to increasing concerns about the practice. Brothels were closed in a number of European cities and prostitutes were often punished harshly. But prostitution continued to exist, and some came to see it as a necessary evil. In some jurisdictions, particularly from the late eighteenth century on, it was decided that regulating prostitution was a better policy than trying to eliminate it. Concerns about the threat of venereal disease, especially to military personnel, played a significant role in this development. "Licensed" houses of prostitution were established, with regular medical examination of the prostitutes in an effort to control venereal disease. For example, Berlin set up a system of regulated prostitution in the 1790s. In Paris, the regulation of prostitution began around the turn of the nineteenth century, and continued well into the twentieth century.[32]

Mary Spongberg has argued that in the nineteenth century, venereal disease came to be more and more associated with prostitutes (and, by extension, with women of "loose morals"). Although it was believed by doctors that any woman, even a virgin, could transmit venereal disease, the prostitute became the obvious symbol of sexual excess and the easiest target for regulation. As Spongberg noted, it was impossible to police all women, and "virtuous" women would have been outraged at the idea that they were diseased. Blame was thus increasingly shifted specifically toward prostitutes. Spongberg wrote that "[p]rostitutes were seen as both physically and morally responsible for the spread of venereal disease. They were seen not merely as agents of transmission but as inherently diseased, if not the disease itself."[33]

This view harmonized with the Victorian idea that most women were innately pure and relatively free of sexual desire. Women who could not control their sexuality were treated as pathological. These women appeared to have a particular "aptitude" for prostitution, according to medical opinion. In spite of the condemnation of prostitution, many in Victorian society believed that it served a useful purpose. Prostitution provided an avenue where men could relieve their "uncontrollable" sexual urges. Young men not in a position to marry, for example, could rely on a prostitute to satisfy their sexual desires, without "ruining" a respectable woman or resorting to the "abominable" vice of masturbation. Although infidelity in married men was not officially condoned, there were those who implicitly accepted the fact that prostitution also provided an outlet for a husband with strong sexual desires to spare his wife unwanted sex.[34]

The idea of quarantining prostitutes with venereal disease while they underwent treatment for their condition was first voiced in the early days of syphilis. Torella, who had been one of the first to claim that men are more likely to catch syphilis from women than vice versa, called at the end of the fifteenth century for the inspection of

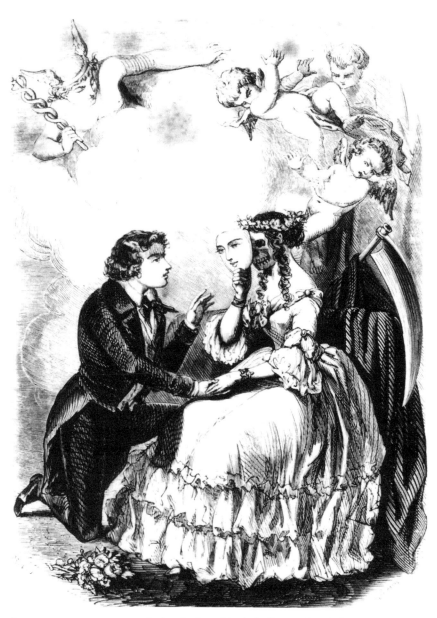

A young man woos a woman, who has the face of death (indicating that she has syphilis) behind her mask. From Auguste Marseille Barthëmely, *Syphilis: poëme en quatre chants* (Paris, 1851) [Courtesy of the National Library of Medicine].

prostitutes and the forced detention of those who were infected until they had fully recovered.[35] Although this demand was not implemented at the time, the practice of isolating women with venereal disease was later adopted in various locales. In the sixteenth century, for example, the Italian city-state of Venice developed institutions for the confinement of certain types of women in part as a response to the spread of syphilis. Although it is true that both men and women were frequently treated in special hospitals established for syphilitics in Italy (and elsewhere as well), it was only "fallen women" who were encouraged to repent and to enter a convent designed for repentant prostitutes. While this convent was designed to "save" women who had already fallen into a life of vice and disease, the Venetians took the concept a step further by founding another institution to protect beautiful young girls before they had an opportunity to suffer such a fate. The so-called *Zitrelle* was a house of refuge that required the girls who were admitted to be beautiful. It was based on the premise that extreme beauty was dangerous. It was believed that very beautiful women also often suffered from sexual excess and that they served as temptresses to men. Thus beautiful girls who were in the most danger of being deflowered were encouraged to enter the *Zitrelle* and remain there until the time of their marriage. Both the convent for repentant prostitutes and the *Zitrelle* were placed on islands to ensure their physical remoteness, to "quarantine" the women for their own protection and that of the rest of Venetian society.[36]

The regulatory systems for prostitution that were established beginning in the late eighteenth century frequently incorporated some type of quarantine measures. Under the French system, for example, prostitutes who were examined and found to have a venereal disease were required to undergo a course of treatment at a prison hospital. The 1864 British law that established a system of regulated prostitution in naval ports and garrison towns gave magistrates the authority to order the detention of a diseased woman for up to three months.[37] In Italy, prostitutes could also be required to undergo treatment if infected. A decree in 1862 established hospitals with the characteristics of prisons for the treatment of prostitutes with venereal disease. Of these Italian hospitals, Bruno Wanrooij has written, "The women, who were essentially locked up, were obliged to work and were not allowed to have contacts with the outside world without permission of the director. They were subject to strict discipline and in the case of any infraction of the rules, risked punishments such as the reduction of food rations."[38] Infected prostitutes in Paris were also frequently confined to a hospital that was much like a prison.[39]

Abolitionists, who wished to eliminate prostitution, were opposed to the system of regulation, which they saw as giving legal sanction to the practice. They argued that regulation did not ensure that venereal disease would not spread, since medical examination could not always detect syphilis. Prostitutes who appeared to be healthy could still be infected with the disease. In addition, abolitionists attacked the "double standard" that excused men who engaged in illicit sex because of their supposed "uncontrollable" sex drive and penalized only women. Why, they asked, was attention focused only on prostitutes, and not on male clients who could equally well infect a prostitute? Infection was a two-way street. In addition, abolitionists pointed out that the responsibility for "innocent victims" of syphilis, women who caught the disease from their husbands and children who were born infected, could not be laid at the feet of prostitutes. Rather it was the male clients who served as the intermediaries in transmitting the disease to their families. As for the argument that prostitutes were largely patronized by young single men seeking sexual release, various studies suggested that the typical customer of a prostitute was more likely a married man of mature years.[40] Concerns were also expressed by some about the curtailment of civil liberties involved in forcing prostitutes to undergo examination and treatment for venereal disease.[41] Abolitionists did succeed in having the regulation ordinances repealed in England and Norway late in the nineteenth century, but the system of licensed prostitution continued on into the twentieth century in many European countries.[42]

Two aspects of syphilis that did specifically involve women were the congenital form of the disease and transmission of the disease from a woman to a baby or vice versa during breast feeding. From almost the time of recognition of the disease, the two-way transmission of the disease between a mother or wet nurse and a baby was recognized. As early as 1497, for example, Torella described the symptoms of syphilis in a suckling infant and suggested that the baby acquired the disease from an infected wet nurse (or presumably an infected mother if she were nursing her own baby, but Torella may have hesitated to blame a mother). He noted that in these children the disease first appeared in the mouth or on the face, where the baby was in contact with the woman's breast. Torella may have specifically had in mind transmission of the disease through contact of the baby with a syphilitic sore on the woman, but others later recognized that the disease could be transmitted through the milk of the mother or wet nurse. It was also known early on that a syphilitic infant could transmit the disease to the wet nurse. If the baby had a syphilitic sore on its mouth, constant contact with the breast of the wet nurse could lead to infection of the woman.[43]

Physicians also recognized that the baby of an infected mother might acquire the disease while in the womb or while passing through the birth canal. We now know that the microorganism that causes syphilis can cross the placenta from mother to baby at any time during pregnancy, or the baby can be infected during labor or delivery. This type of infection is known as congenital syphilis. Syphilis can lead to a miscarriage or stillbirth or medical complications at or after birth, such as an inflammation of the cornea that can cause blindness. Similarly, the syphilis microorganism can be transmitted in the breast milk.

It was also commonly believed that syphilis can be inherited. Most physicians accepted the idea that in addition to a fetus acquiring the disease from the mother in the womb or during birth, it could also be infected by the father at the moment of conception, a view that we reject today. In the late nineteenth and early twentieth centuries, when Europeans and Americans became obsessed with concerns over "degeneration" of the race (as will be discussed in the next chapter), there was widespread concern about the effects of "hereditary syphilis."[44] The noted syphilologist, Alfred Fournier, for example, wrote in 1904:

> It emerges from recent research that syphilis can, because of its hereditary consequences, debase and corrupt the species by producing inferior, decadent, dystrophic and deficient beings. Yes, deficient; they can be physically deficient . . . or they can be mentally deficient, being, according to the degree of their intellectual debasement, retarded, simple-minded, unbalanced, insane, imbecilic or idiotic.[45]

It was not until after World War II that the idea that syphilis could be inherited, i.e., actually passed down through the genes, was completely disproved. A child born with syphilis can have acquired the infection only from a syphilitic mother (e.g., by the microorganisms that cause the disease crossing the placenta). Syphilis, in other words, can be congenital (from birth), but is not hereditary. Congenital syphilis can now be prevented if an infected mother is treated with antibiotics early enough in her pregnancy.[46]

Wet nursing became popular with European women of the upper and middle classes, who tended to prefer not to nurse their babies, by the seventeenth century. In addition, wet nurses were needed to feed the large numbers of abandoned children in foundling homes, and in these cases it was often not known for certain whether or not the mother was infected. Most of the wet nurses, not surprisingly, came from the poorer classes and often from rural areas. As this was before the development of pasteurization for milk and of baby formulas, babies who were fed on the milk of cows or other animals suffered a much higher mortality rate than those who were breast-fed. Systems of regulations were developed to try to ensure that woman who served as wet nurses did not have syphilis and that syphilitic infants were not given to wet nurses for breast feeding. However, since there was no definitive test available for syphilis, a disease that could be especially difficult to detect in the early weeks of the life of a newborn, these procedures did not eliminate the transmission of the disease by breastfeeding.[47]

Even as late as the turn of the twentieth century, the contraction of syphilis through wet nursing of foundlings was still a significant problem. One paper read at the meeting of the American Medical Association in 1906, for example, called the wet nursing of foundlings "a pernicious practice" since it could lead to the infection of the nurse with syphilis, and she might then pass the disease on to her husband and unborn children. Although recognizing that many of the babies would die without wet nursing, the author complained that the babies were saved "at the terrible cost of syphilizing an innocent woman and her child." He was thankful, however, that the wet nursing of foundlings had not gained much of a foothold in the United States, as contrasted with Europe.[48]

David Kertzer has recently published a fascinating account of the story of one of these wet nurses, entitled *Amalia's Tale: A Poor Peasant, an Ambitious Attorney, and a Fight for Justice*. Amalia was one of the many poor village women in Italy in the late nineteenth century who hired herself out as a wet nurse for a foundling home, in this case in the city of Bologna. She was given an infant to take home and nurse. The child appeared to be sick, and Amalia asked to be given another baby instead, but the foundling home insisted that she take the one that they had selected for her. Amalia contracted syphilis from the child, and then infected her husband. She also later had several children who were born dead or died soon after birth. An ambitious young attorney, seeking to make his mark in the world, took up her cause and sued the foundling home on her behalf, although it seemed very unlikely that a poor peasant woman could prevail in court over a foundling home that was supported by the gentry of Bologna. Although Amalia remarkably won her case, after some ten years and after several appeals, her victory was a somewhat hollow one, for the money that she was awarded was completely eaten up by lawyer's fees and other expenses incurred in pursuing the case.[49]

WHAT'S IN A NAME?

As we have seen, syphilis had many names during its early history, including the French disease, the great pox, and *morbus venerus*. The term *lues venereal* (venereal disease) also came into frequent use from the late sixteenth century on.[50] But how did the disease acquire its modern name? The word "syphilis" was introduced by the Italian physician Girolamo Fracastoro in his *Syphilis sive morbus gallicus*, a long poem in Latin published in 1530. This extremely popular work was published in more than one hundred editions over the course of the sixteenth century. The poem tells the story of a shepherd named Syphilus. The shepherd kept the flocks of a king named Alcithous. One year the animals perished for lack of water, and an angry Syphilus blasphemed the Sun-God and overturned his altars. He pledged from that day forth to worship only King Alcithous. The enraged Sun-God visited a new disease on the inhabitants of the land as punishment, with Syphilus being the first victim.[51] Fracastoro wrote that:

> He first wore buboes dreadful to the sight,
> First felt strange pains and sleepless past the night;
> From him the malady received its name.[52]

Fracastoro was born in Verona, Italy, about 1480 (dates of his birth are given in various sources as from 1478 to 1483). He was a fellow student of the great astronomer Copernicus, who postulated that the earth revolved about the sun, at the University of Padua, where he studied philosophy and medicine. The derivation of the name "Syphilis" by Fracastoro is unknown, but many scholars regard the name (often spelled Syphilus) as a medieval form of Sipylus, a character in the poem *Metamorphoses* by the classical Roman poet Ovid.[53]

Fracastoro's mythical explanation of the origins of syphilis was not meant to be taken literally. In the poem, he introduced a naturalistic explanation for the spread of disease that he was to expand upon in a later, more scholarly work. To explain the transmission of syphilis, Fracastoro used the concept of "seeds" (*semina*). These particles are responsible for carrying the disease for one person to another, i.e., for the contagion of syphilis. It should be clearly understood, however, that Fracastoro's concept of seeds of contagion was by no means a forerunner of the modern germ theory of disease. He could hardly have been thinking in terms of his "seeds" being microorganisms, as these organisms had not yet even been discovered, nor had the microscope been invented at the time he published his work. Rather, his seeds were imperceptible particles that were spontaneously generated during certain types of putrefaction. He also did not rule out the possibility that the production of poisonous seeds was somehow sparked by certain planetary conjunctions in the heavens.[54]

In spite of the popularity of Fracastoro's poem, the name syphilis did not immediately replace other terms for the disease. It was scarcely used at all before the end of the eighteenth century, and did not become the predominant term for describing the disease until the nineteenth century.[55]

While on the subject of names, one can note that many famous individuals have had, or are suspected of having had, syphilis. Those for whom the evidence of the disease seems definitive include the composer Robert Schumann, the writers Gustave Flaubert and Guy de Maupassant, the artist Paul Gauguin, and the gangster Al Capone. Some authors have speculated that Ludwig van Beethoven, Friedrich Nietzsche, Oscar Wilde, Vincent van Gogh, Adolf Hitler, and even Abraham Lincoln and his wife may have suffered from syphilis, but the evidence is not conclusive in these cases. Deborah Hayden has discussed famous syphilitics and possible syphilitics in depth in her book *Pox: Genius, Madness, and the Mysteries of Syphilis*.[56]

TREATMENT

Once the venereal nature of syphilis was understood, people could be (and were) warned against having intimate relations with individuals who were infected, assuming they could identify the infected. But once one had contracted the disease, what remedies were available to alleviate, if not cure, the malady? Some of those who believed that the pox was the just rewards of immoral behavior questioned whether or not those afflicted with the disease even deserved to be treated.[57]

Not surprisingly, when this terrible new disease first appeared, all sorts of remedies were recommended for dealing with it. For example, Torella advised such strange treatments as applying a cock or pigeon flayed alive, or a live frog cut in two, to an infected penis.[58] A major aim of most treatment was to remove the morbid matter causing the disease from the patient. This could be done in various ways, for example, by blood-letting or the use of laxatives. An alternative method involved having the patient bathe in a mixture of wine and herbs, or in olive oil. Syphilitics could also be placed in an enclosed heated space, causing them to sweat, another mechanism for eliminating corrupt matter from the body.[59]

The two remedies that eventually came to be by far the most popular, however, were mercury and guaiacum. Mercury had long been used, especially by the Arabs, in the treatment of skin diseases and even leprosy. Therefore it seemed reasonable to try it against syphilis, which generally involved skin lesions and was thought to resemble leprosy. Numerous physicians in the early sixteenth century advocated the use of mercury in the forms of ointments or rubs. Even antivenereal underpants, coated on the inside with a mercurial ointment, were available in Italy. It was recognized, however, that excess mercury could be harmful. Overdosing with mercury could lead to such toxic side effects as shaking, paralysis, and the loosening and loss of teeth. Sometimes the mercury was applied to the body and the patient was then placed in a heated area for long periods of time. This introduced the possibility of mercury vapors entering the respiratory tract, which could be very dangerous.[60]

At first mercury was only given externally, for example, in the form of an ointment. The internal administration of mercury seemed to be too dangerous. At the end of the eighteenth century, however, the internal administration of mercury began to overtake the external methods. The mercury could be administered in the form of enemas, or taken orally in a gum form or as calomel (the salt mercurous chloride). Van Swieten's liquor, consisting of grains of corrosive sublimate (mercuric chloride) dissolved in a solution of water and alcohol, became popular in the late eighteenth century. Mercury poisoning was probably not uncommon, but side effects that were probably due to the treatment were often attributed to the disease itself. Mercury remained the preferred treatment for syphilis up into the twentieth century.[61]

The principal challenger to mercury in the early history of syphilis was guaiacum (or guaiac) wood. The guaiacum tree was native to the Indies, and the Spanish and the Portuguese began using the wood to treat syphilis by the early fifteenth century. At the time, it was widely believed that God often placed remedies for a disease in the areas where that disease flourished. Since many Europeans began to ascribe the origins of syphilis to the Americas, it did not seem unreasonable that a cure for the disease might exist in that part of the world.[62]

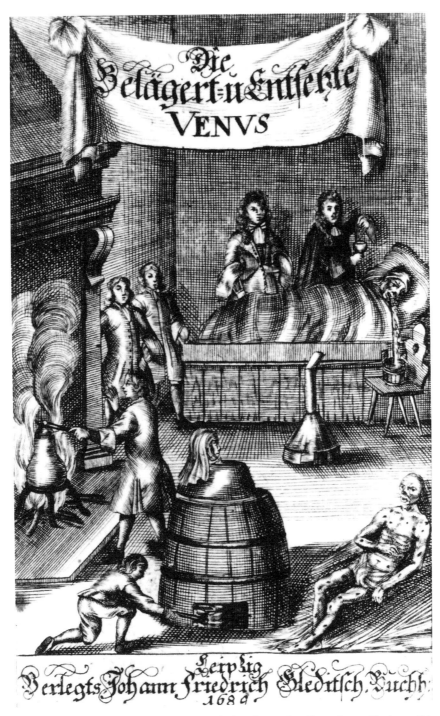

Various methods of treatment for syphilis, including fumigation. From Steven Blankaart, *Die belägert- und entsetzte Venus* (Augsburg, 1710) [Courtesy of the National Library of Medicine].

The wood was administered by grinding it into a powder and then boiling it in water. The resulting decoction (the liquid remaining when the wood is removed) was then ingested by the patient. But typically treatment with guaiacum involved much more than simply drinking a decoction made from the wood. The patient was generally placed in a warm room and put on a strict diet with limited food intake. He or she was also given mild laxatives. The patient then drank a large dose of the decoction daily, after which he or she was wrapped in blankets to induce sweating. This regimen was carried out for thirty days, and was undoubtedly quite debilitating to the patient. A 1519 book by the German humanist and religious reformer Ulrich von Hutten on guaiacum, which was translated into several languages, helped to popularize the drug. Hutten himself suffered from syphilis and was convinced that he had been cured by guaiacum (although he appears to have eventually died of syphilis). As someone who was opposed to the medical establishment, he was delighted to recommend an empirical remedy that came from a "barbarian" land with no doctors.[63]

Historian Sheldon Watts has suggested that the Spaniard Oviedo, whom we have already encountered as the first person to ascribe the origins of syphilis to the New World, helped to popularize guaiacum for financial reasons. While in the Indies, Oviedo learned that the wood was a reputed cure for syphilis. According to Watts, Oviedo knew that the public accepted the doctrine that for every disease or poison God had placed a cure nearby, and so he claimed that the people of the Indies had long suffered from syphilis but were able to cure the disease with guaiacum. He arranged for his partners, the Fugger family of bankers, to obtain monopoly rights from the King of Spain to import and market the wood throughout the Spanish Empire. This arrangement resulted in handsome profits for Oviedo and the Fuggers.[64]

Mercury and guaiacum were also not infrequently used together in the treatment of syphilitics by doctors anxious to cover all bases. In the sixteenth century, the efficacy of guaiacum was challenged by Paracelsus, and its use began to progressively decline. Sometimes it was replaced by other woods and roots, included sarsaparilla, another American import. Mercury temporarily lost some of its credibility around the beginning of the nineteenth century, but made a comeback by the 1860s. Although there were certain new treatments that were employed in the nineteenth century, such as potassium iodide and certain preparations of arsenic, Quétel has concluded that other forms of treatment had a hard time competing with mercury. Mercury remained king in the treatment of syphilis until the twentieth century, although it left much to be desired as a remedy.[65]

SCIENTIFIC DEVELOPMENTS

Although the medical understanding of syphilis increased over the centuries since its introduction, treatment did not change much and the specific cause of the disease remained unknown until the beginning of the twentieth century. The development of the germ theory of disease by Louis Pasteur in France and Robert Koch in Germany in the period of the 1860s through the 1880s eventually opened the door to important breakthroughs with respect to the disease. The acceptance of the germ theory, which postulated that microorganisms were the cause of infectious disease, led medical researchers to search for the specific pathogenic organisms that were the cause of individual diseases. For example, the microorganism that causes gonorrhea was isolated in 1879 and the one that causes tuberculosis was isolated in 1882.[66]

Understanding the microorganisms that caused specific diseases also led to more systematic efforts to find ways of preventing and curing these diseases. For example, in the late nineteenth and early twentieth centuries, vaccines were developed for the immunization of persons against diseases such as rabies, anthrax, and typhoid. At the time that the germ theory was being established, a procedure for immunizing individuals against one disease, smallpox, already existed. This procedure had been discovered empirically before any knowledge that the disease was caused by a microorganism.

For centuries the practice of inoculating a person with smallpox had been carried out in certain Eastern countries such as China and Turkey. Recognizing that people who contracted smallpox and survived were apparently immune from the disease for the rest of their lives, some individuals began actually trying to cause a mild case of the disease in healthy people as a preventive against their developing a full-blown case of smallpox at a later date. A common means of carrying out the procedure was by dipping a needle into a pustule (pimple containing pus) on the body of a smallpox victim, and then scratching the arm of a healthy individual. Sometimes other methods were used, such as blowing a powder made from a dried smallpox scab up the nose of the healthy person. This process is known as inoculation. In most cases, the person inoculated developed a relatively mild case of the disease and acquired an immunity to it. Sometimes, however, the inoculated individual contracted a serious case of smallpox, and a very small percentage actually died from the disease.

Smallpox inoculation was introduced into Europe and America in the early eighteenth century. At the end of that century, however, English physician Edward Jenner introduced into medicine the safer procedure that came to be known as vaccination. Jenner's discovery was based on the common folk belief of the day that milkmaids who acquired a disease known as cowpox from cows seemed to be immune to smallpox. In order to determine whether or not cowpox actually protected against smallpox, Jenner inoculated a young boy with fluid from a cowpox sore on the arm of a milkmaid in 1796. When Jenner later tried to inoculate the boy with smallpox, the boy proved to be immune. Jenner performed other successful trials, and two years later published a book on the subject. To distinguish his procedure, which involved the use of cowpox, from inoculation with smallpox itself, Jenner called it vaccination (from the Latin word for cow, *vacca*). In time, the procedure came to be widely accepted and employed, although not without controversy.[67]

The example of inoculation and vaccination against smallpox served as a stimulus and model to encourage others to try to develop a method of immunization against syphilis, even though the cause of this disease was also not known at the time. The first person to have attempted such a procedure would appear to have been the French physician Joseph-Alexandre Auzias-Turenne. Researchers had been having difficulty producing syphilis in animals, thus inhibiting experimentation on the disease. Some scientists concluded that the disease could not be reproduced in animals, but Auzias-Turenne disagreed with this view. He claimed in 1844 that he had successfully transmitted syphilis to monkeys by inoculating them with pus from a chancre (a lesion on the skin commonly produced in syphilis) of a person infected with the disease. Furthermore, he showed that with repeated inoculation of the monkeys with syphilis, the size of the lesion or chancre produced in the monkey progressively decreased, so that eventually inoculation produced no lesion at all. Auzias-Turenne concluded that the monkeys had become immunized against syphilis so that further inoculations produced no new symptoms. He referred to this process as "syphilization."

Not everyone was convinced that Auzias-Turenne had indeed successfully immunized monkeys against syphilis, but he proceeded to try the procedure in clinical studies. Mostly he worked with syphilitic prostitutes. He believed that syphilization could be used as a preventative against the disease, by producing immunity, and even suggested that it might be in the general interest to apply the procedure to all prostitutes. Although many of Auzias-Turenne's colleagues challenged his views, for a time the practice of syphilization continued to gain new advocates. Casimir Sperino of the Hospital for Venereal Women in Turin, Italy, for example, syphilized fifty-two women and reported that not only did they fail to develop constitutional syphilis after more than five months of observation, but their health actually improved. He argued for the use of the procedure as a treatment for those infected with syphilis as well as a preventative. Once again we see women, especially prostitutes, singled out as a source of transmission of syphilis. Carl Wilhelm Boeck in Oslo, Norway, also experimented with and championed syphilization. By the late 1860s, however, evidence was accumulating that syphilization did not work either as a cure or preventative for syphilis, and the practice eventually disappeared. The ethics of many of these syphilization experiments is problematic since they were usually performed on unwilling, or at least uninformed, subjects (for example, hospitalized prostitutes, soldiers, and even infants).[68]

It is not surprising that in a period before it had been established that infectious diseases are caused by microorganisms the search for a vaccine against syphilis was unsuccessful. By the early 1890s, the German bacteriologist Albert Neisser, who had discovered the bacillus that caused gonorrhea, was able to apply the new knowledge of microorganisms to an attempt to develop a syphilis vaccine. He tested his experimental vaccine, prepared from the blood serum of people infected with syphilis, on several young girls and female prostitutes. Apparently he did not obtain the permission of the subjects or their legal guardians, and the experiments eventually led to attacks against Neisser and his criminal prosecution. He was convicted and fined three hundred marks, although Susan Lederer has pointed out that anti-Semitism may have played a role in these court proceedings. Another result of this case was that the Prussian government issued a directive that prohibited medical experimentation on humans without their consent.[69]

In the first decade of the twentieth century, Elie Metchnikoff and Emile Roux at the Pasteur Institute in Paris demonstrated that they could transmit syphilis to chimpanzees using human-infected material. They also showed they could transmit the disease from one chimpanzee to another. Next they experimented to see whether an ointment of calomel, a mercury compound frequently used in an effort to treat syphilis, could prevent the development of syphilis lesions in the animals. The results seemed promising, suggesting that perhaps routine treatment with calomel following exposure to syphilis could prevent the disease from developing. A medical student in Paris read about their experiments and convinced Metchnikoff and Roux to experiment on him. On January 23, 1906, infectious material from a syphilitic chancre was inoculated onto the student's penis. The site was rubbed with calomel and the student was examined periodically by a physician over the next several months with no evidence of the appearance of syphilis. The procedure was controversial, however, and one case hardly constituted proof of success. Metchnikoff and Roux did not follow up on this work, which was soon overshadowed by Paul Ehrlich's discovery of the antisyphilitic drug Salvarsan in 1910.[70]

In 1905, the German zoologist Fritz Schaudinn and syphilologist Erich Hoffman isolated a microorganism from a syphilitic patient. Soon they had obtained the organism from eleven patients and were able to show that it was clearly the cause of the disease. Schaudinn called the organism *Treponema* (because it resembled a twisted thread) *palladium* (because of its pale color). It was also commonly known as *Spirochaeta pallida*, and came to be called a spirochete in popular usage. Although the news of this discovery was initially viewed with skepticism in some quarters, Schaudinn and Hoffman's results were quickly confirmed by others. Finally the cause of syphilis was understood.[71]

Within two years of the discovery of the syphilis organism, the German bacteriologist August von Wasserman developed the first blood test for the detection of syphilis. The Wasserman test was extremely effective in identifying early syphilis, but was less useful in the later stages of the disease because it produced a high percentage of false negatives. Later variations of the Wasserman test made it more reliable. The test became routine for cases of suspected syphilis.[72]

Thus in the early years of the twentieth century the cause of syphilis was uncovered and a diagnostic test for its detection became available. Soon another major advance occurred, this one also in Germany (which was the leading nation in medical research at the time), that was to transform the treatment of the disease. Paul Ehrlich, who had been devoting much of his research in the 1890s to immunology, returned in the first decade of the twentieth century to a subject that had interested him earlier, the development of chemical agents to treat infectious disease. Ehrlich and his coworkers in Frankfurt began a search for chemical substances that would attack disease-causing microorganisms within the body. The hope was to find chemical drugs that acted like "magic bullets" that would specifically destroy the microorganisms without injury to human cells. His work initially focused on a group of microorganisms called trypanosomes, which caused such diseases as sleeping sickness.

Ehrlich learned in 1905 that two British researchers had found that the arsenic-containing organic compound atoxyl could eliminate trypanosomes from the blood of infected animals. Unfortunately, it was soon found that relapses commonly occurred and that that the large therapeutic doses required could damage the optic nerve and produce blindness. Ehrlich reasoned, however, that he might be able to modify the structure of atoxyl in a way that reduced or eliminated its effect on the optic nerve while still retaining its toxicity toward trypanosomes. Over the next few years, hundreds of arsenic compounds were synthesized and tested in his laboratory.

After the discovery of the spirochete that caused syphilis in 1905, Ehrlich began trying arsenical drugs against syphilis as well because there appeared to be a similarity between trypanosomes and spirochetes. In 1909, the Japanese scientist Sahachiro Hata, working in Ehrlich's laboratory, discovered that compound number 606 was effective in treating syphilis infections in rabbits. After extensive animal tests, Ehrlich arranged for the drug to be distributed to selected medical specialists for human clinical trials. The results were promising, and in 1910 Ehrlich announced the new drug to the world. Demand for 606 soon outgrew the ability of Ehrlich's laboratory to prepare it, and he arranged with a German chemical company to produce the drug under the tradename Salvarsan.[73]

Salvarsan represented the first effective treatment for syphilis, and hence was hailed as a major medical breakthrough. Although the drug was indeed a major advance in the treatment of the disease, it was by no means an ideal therapeutic agent. Salvarsan, as an arsenical compound, had serious side effects. It also had to be administered by injection, and treatment was prolonged, sometimes involving an injection a week for a year or more. Ehrlich did introduce a somewhat improved form of the drug, Neosalvarsan, within a few years, and other arsenicals were introduced later. In spite of the problems with arsenical therapy, it remained the primary form of treatment of syphilis from its introduction until the discovery of the effectiveness of penicillin against the disease in the 1940s.

TWO

A "SECRET DISEASE": SYPHILIS IN AMERICA BEFORE THE FIRST WORLD WAR

THE COLONIAL PERIOD

Whether or not syphilis was present in America before the arrival of Columbus, it was clearly established there in the colonial period, both among the colonists and the native peoples. Syphilis was common in Europe at the time, and undoubtedly some of the explorers, settlers, and others traveling to the New World carried the disease with them. There were sexual relations between some of the colonists and the natives, so the disease could be transmitted between the two populations. Little information is available about syphilis in the early period of colonization, but scattered reports do indicate its presence in the colonies at an early date.

On Columbus' second voyage to America in late 1493, he established a colony with over a thousand residents on the island of Hispaniola (today occupied by Haiti and the Dominican Republic). On his next voyage in 1498, he found that many of the settlers had died and many of the survivors suffered from various illnesses, including apparently syphilis.[1] Only the Spanish (and to some extent the Portuguese in Brazil) had an extensive and organized colonial empire in the Americas in the sixteenth century. It is not surprising then that the earliest reports of syphilis as a problem in America came from New Spain. In 1539, for example, a separate hospital was built exclusively for syphilis patients near the City of Mexico. By 1569, reports indicate that physicians at the Hospital de Santa Cruz, about fifty miles from the City of Mexico, were using native herbs to treat syphilis and other diseases.[2]

The story of the British North American colonies that were to evolve into the United States begins with the settlement of Jamestown, Virginia, in 1607. Excavation of two seventeenth-century burial sites inside the perimeter of James Fort has provided evidence that syphilis was present at Jamestown. One of the skeletons excavated revealed signs of tertiary syphilis. Interestingly, the body was that of a young man of African descent, one of several bodies of African ancestry found at this site. Africans, both slaves and free men, accompanied Europeans on exploration and colonization voyages from the early days of the New World discovery, and were living in Jamestown at least by 1624. It is not known whether this particular man contracted the disease before or after he arrived in Jamestown. Given the fact that he had tertiary syphilis, he must have been suffering from the disease for a number of years at the time of his death, which was caused by a gunshot wound to the head.[3]

As more colonies were established and grew in size, reports of the disease became more common. A minor syphilis outbreak occurred in Boston in 1646. John Winthrop, the first governor of the Massachusetts colony, recorded that the disease had been brought into Boston by a cooper (barrel maker) who had worked on a ship. He in turn gave syphilis to his wife, and the disease eventually spread to fifteen neighbors.[4] As urban populations increased and cities became more sophisticated in the American colonies, commercialized vice, such as prostitution, also increased. By the early eighteenth century, there were several houses of prostitution in both Boston and Philadelphia.[5] Increased sexual freedom and prostitution probably contributed to a rise in the incidence of venereal disease. In the early 1700s, the famous Boston cleric Cotton Mather, who had earlier decried the presence of houses of prostitution in the city, complained about the many who were afflicted with syphilis. He referred to it as a "secret disease," and noted that death records frequently reported it covertly under the term "consumption" (which generally meant tuberculosis).[6] A colonial almanac from 1734 also noted that young men from the colonies who visited London frequently returned with a venereal disease.[7]

Sex between the settlers and the Indians, including intermarriage, was not uncommon, and venereal disease was transmitted both ways. Some travel narratives of the eighteenth century warned readers that venereal disease was common in many tribes. Of course, these accounts may well have been colored by the tendency of white settlers to disapprove of the generally more open sexuality of the Indians. Other accounts of the period describe examples of Indians contracting venereal diseases from traders.[8] Indian women were seen by many colonial men as wild, passionate, and alluring. As early as 1631, a young man was ordered to be whipped by the Massachusetts General Court for seducing an Indian woman. A number of cases of fornication involving colonists and Indians appeared on the court docket of Plymouth Colony over the years, almost all of which involved a white male initiating sex with an Indian woman. There was at least one case, however, in which a female colonist was whipped for seducing an Indian man.[9]

Syphilis was apparently introduced into the California Indian population by Hispanic settlers in the latter part of the eighteenth century. Colonists, probably especially soldiers, sometimes raped Indian women, who became infected and passed the disease on to others in the tribe.[10] Missionaries knew that syphilis was common among California Indians by the early nineteenth century. The disease in pregnant women was probably responsible for many spontaneous abortions, stillbirths, and birth defects in the Indian population.[11] However, compared to the devastation caused by other European diseases, such as smallpox, the damage inflicted on the Indian population by syphilis was relatively small. The impact of the new diseases from Europe on the Indians, who had no natural immunity to these infections to which they had not been exposed before, constituted, in the words of Colin Calloway, "one of the greatest biological catastrophes in history." Some tribes were essentially completely wiped out, while others lost 50 percent or more of their population.[12]

In what might be thought of as an early example of germ warfare, British soldiers or settlers have been accused of giving Indians blankets that had deliberately been infected with smallpox, although the evidence for these charges is not definitive. There is adequate documentation, however, that such a plan was seriously contemplated on at least one occasion. In a similar vein, the Governor of the Louisiana territory suggested in 1724 a mechanism that would allow him to deal with the problem of "human debris" that had emigrated from Paris, as well as with the Indian population. He claimed that the territory included a number of "useless" women who were infected with syphilis and responsible for "ruining" sailors. He proposed that these women be sent "into the interior" to live with the Indians, where they would presumably spread the disease among the natives. It is not clear, however, that this proposal was ever carried out.[13]

Sexual relations, whether consensual or not, between white men and black slaves were also common, so that syphilis became entrenched in the African American population as well. Female slaves were not infrequently raped by their masters. Todd Savitt, in his study of medicine and slavery in antebellum Virginia, found a significant number of references in the case books of physicians to the treatment of syphilis and gonorrhea among both blacks and whites. Indentured servants were also at risk of being sexually exploited. Young female servants were especially vulnerable to sexual advances by their masters.[14] One colonist, Richard More, recorded that when he visited the home of Joseph Wickes in Patuxent, Maryland, in 1656, he found that Wickes' new servant, Anne Gould, was suffering so badly from syphilis that she could barely walk. Apparently she contracted the disease when she was raped by her former master, Richard Owens. The court simply ignored the rape, but did order Owens to provide Wicks, who was seen as the victim of fraud, with another servant.[15]

Medical historian John Duffy has argued that the American colonies were relatively free of venereal disease, at least in the early colonial period, because there are so few references to these ailments in colonial records. Noting that the colonists, even the

Puritans, were not as prudish as sometimes portrayed, he argues that they would not have hesitated to discuss the subject (at least with reference to others) in their private correspondence and diaries. Duffy conceded that the incidence of such diseases likely increased somewhat following the French and Indian War (1756–1763), a result of the presence of large numbers of European soldiers and the social and moral disruptions caused by the war. He notes, for example, that there was a considerable increase in advertisements for venereal disease cures in colonial newspapers by the 1760s.[16]

Certainly by the late eighteenth century venereal disease was seen as a problem in the larger cities of North America, particularly in seaports such as Boston, New York, Philadelphia, and Charleston. At the time, Philadelphia was the largest city on the continent, and probably allowed the greatest degree of personal, including sexual, freedom. With the relative lack of restraint in the sexual climate came a high venereal disease rate, involving both syphilis and gonorrhea. In the Pennsylvania Hospital, the nation's oldest such institution, patients with venereal disease were placed in separate wards from the main building. Of those entering the almshouse in Philadelphia at the end of the century, about 10 percent were infected with venereal disease. Some of the infants brought to or born in the almshouse also had venereal infections. Mariners and prostitutes were among the most common of the almshouse patients, often leaving before having fully recovered and thus further spreading the disease.[17]

War has traditionally provided a stimulus to the spread of venereal disease. Oscar Reiss has noted that "[s]yphilis and armies were like Hansel and Gretel. They went into the unknown hand-in-hand."[18] It is thus likely that the incidence of syphilis rose during the American Revolutionary War. Soldiers were away from the restraints of home and family, and the troops frequently attracted prostitutes. In her history of the Army Medical department, Mary Gillett has pointed out that venereal disease was an ever-present threat to eighteenth-century armies. Disease in general was responsible for vastly more deaths than combat at the time. An estimated 90 percent of deaths in the Continental Army and 84 percent of deaths in the British Army were due to disease in the American Revolution. Gillett documents that venereal disease, including syphilis, was not infrequently seen among the troops in the army hospitals of the time. In August of 1777, for example, there were fourteen cases of syphilis in the army hospital at Albany, New York. In the summer of 1782, 38 of the approximately 225 patients at the army hospital in New Windsor, New York, were suffering from venereal disease, apparently the most common ailment in the facility at the time. In the battle for New York, George Washington complained about the number of his troops who were unfit for duty because of venereal disease.[19]

The incidence of venereal disease was probably greater than the records show because it was not always reported. Victims of the disease in the military were frequently punished and thus sometimes tried to hide the ailment. In fact, the Continental Congress, desperate for money to supply the army, even tried to use venereal disease as a fund-raising device. In January 1778, the Congress resolved that every officer hospitalized with venereal disease should be fined $10 and every soldier $4, with the proceeds going to the purchase of blankets and shirts for the troops.[20]

FROM REPUBLIC TO REBELLION

With the signing of the Treaty of Paris in 1783, the Revolutionary War came to an end and the United States entered upon its existence as a sovereign nation. As the new republic entered the nineteenth century, venereal disease continued to pose a threat to public health. Statistics adequate to allow one to assess the scale of the problem do not exist, and Americans of the period were frequently hesitant to openly discuss sexually transmitted diseases. As Gerald Grob has commented, "Syphilitic and gonococcal infections were by no means uncommon, even though estimates of their prevalence are problematic."[21] But some information documenting issues surrounding syphilis and other venereal diseases does exist.

As newspapers grew up and spread, the advertisements for various remedies for "secret diseases" increased, as did advertisements from healers who claimed to be able to cure venereal disease. One advertisement in a Philadelphia newspaper in 1797, for example, was for a venereal disease cure called Laffecteur's Specific, which supposedly contained only plant materials and no mercury.[22] Prostitution, seen as a major cause of the spread of venereal disease, also increased. An 1804 article in the *Medical Repository*, the nation's first medical journal, estimated that there were about 2,100 prostitutes in New York City and some 160 "bawdy and dancing-houses." The editor was especially concerned that there was no regulation of prostitution (e.g., no health inspections), and argued that this situation led to the diffusion of venereal disease.[23]

We know that syphilis was one of the medical problems that confronted William Clark and Meriwether Lewis on their 1804–1806 Corps of Discovery expedition, the first step in the westward expansion of the United States. The expedition did not have a doctor, and so medical care had to be provided by the leaders themselves. Lewis, who had substantial frontier experience, was probably aware that syphilis had spread to the Indian populations that they would encounter. The disease had most likely been brought to the plains Indians by traders from Canada in the late nineteenth century. It was undoubtedly widespread in parts of Canada at the time, as a French doctor reported in 1801 that some 5,800 French-Canadians were infected.[24]

The medical supplies carried on the expedition included three remedies used in the treatment of syphilis: calomel (mercurous chloride), Dr. Rush's Bilious Pills (which contained mercury), and a mercury ointment. The former two drugs were administered orally, and the ointment was applied locally to syphilitic lesions or sores. The expedition's list of equipment and drugs also included two items used in the treatment of gonorrhea, the medication copaiba and a penis syringe that was used to inject sugar of lead mixed with water up the urethra.[25]

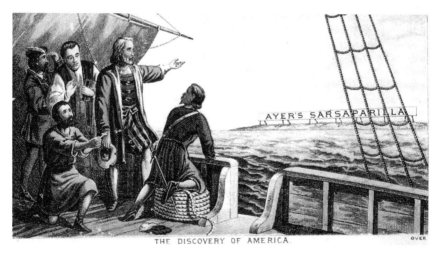

THE DISCOVERY OF AMERICA.

Advertisement for Ayer's Sarsaparilla, nineteenth century. Sarsaparilla was used for the treatment of syphilis because it came from the Americas, where many believed the disease originated. The image of Columbus seeing a sign for the product when he arrived in the New World is intriguing, given that his voyages were frequently blamed for bringing the disease back to Europe [Courtesy of the National Library of Medicine].

Physician-historian Thomas Lowry has published a careful study on the question of venereal disease and the Lewis and Clark expedition. Drawing heavily on the journals of the explorers, Lowry describes the extensive sexual contacts between the members of the expedition and Indian women. In some of the tribes, the explorers record, it was the custom to offer the sexual favors of their women to the white men as a sign of hospitality or as thanks for some gift or favor. Clark noted, for example, that when he successfully treated an ill Indian, the man later returned with his sister and offered her to Clark as a token of gratitude.[26]

Not surprisingly, cases of venereal disease were relatively common among the members of the expedition as a result of this sexual freedom. For example, Lewis recorded using mercury to treat several of his men afflicted with syphilis in the winter of 1806. Although the mercury often appeared to work at first, the disease sometimes resurfaced, which was not uncommon. The obvious symptoms of syphilis can disappear for long stages, thus making it difficult to determine exactly how effective mercury was as a treatment. More likely mercury may have helped to suppress the symptoms of the disease, rather than acting as a cure.[27]

The journals of the explorers record other instances of venereal disease, and Lowry concludes that the evidence suggests "that a considerable number of the men had become infected with syphilis in 1805 and 1806."[28] Lewis himself died in 1809 of gunshot wounds, and it is not entirely clear whether his death was a suicide. Lowry speculates that it is possible that Lewis had contracted syphilis on the expedition, although there is no firm evidence that he engaged in sexual activity on the journey.

If this were the case and his death was a suicide, Lowry concludes that progressive syphilis may have contributed to mental imbalance and depression.[29] Lowry sums up the relationship between venereal disease and the Lewis and Clark expedition as follows:

> Lewis's shopping list shows that he anticipated venereal disease among his men. There is evidence in the records that syphilis was already widespread among the villages that the expedition visited, although whether the Corps brought further venereal disease to the Indians is unknown. There is evidence that there were sexual relations between many of the men of the Corps and some of the Indian women. There is evidence that many, perhaps all, of the men received mercury treatment. . . . In Lewis's tragic death, there is the distinct possibility that syphilis played a part.[30]

Venereal disease continued to be a particular concern in the military. Although little is known about the prevalence of syphilis and gonorrhea in the War of 1812, certain actions taken by the War Office suggest that these infections were seen as a problem. For example, an order was issued that no "noncommissioned officer, musician or soldier of the Army" would receive pay while being treated for a venereal disease, and that the cost of medicines administered would be deducted from his pay. It would appear that this order did not apply to commissioned officers, who were perhaps expected to exhibit greater restraint with respect to sexual activities. Another order stated that women infected with venereal disease should not be allowed to remain with the Army or to draw rations. At least some of the Army surgeons at this time, aware of the toxic side effects of mercury compounds, also began to criticize what they considered to be its careless use to treat syphilis in the field.[31]

Army and civilian physicians, however, still continued to rely heavily upon mercury use in general in the treatment of syphilis. It does appear that the number of cases of venereal disease in the Army declined significantly between 1818 and the beginning of the Civil War. During periods of conflict, however, the numbers would go up. For example, the number of cases of syphilis and gonorrhea increased significantly in Fort Columbus Hospital in New York City between 1839 and 1841, probably due to an influx of injured and sick soldiers who had participated in the Seminole Wars in Florida. In the Mexican War, venereal disease once again became a problem. In June, 1848, for example, the hospital set up by the United States Army in Jalapa, Mexico, had forty-six patients with gonorrhea and thirty-three with primary syphilis.[32]

In civilian life, there was increasing sexual commerce, which most likely contributed to the spread of venereal disease. By the 1830s, D'Emilio and Freedman claim, prostitutes were more visible on the streets of cities than they had been in the eighteenth century, although their numbers were still not large. By the 1850s, however, one report estimated the number of prostitutes in New York City at over 6,000, one for every sixty-four men. Another report from the 1860s estimated the number of brothels in Chicago as over 500. Brothels and other venues where the services of prostitutes could be purchased, such as dance halls, also became more common in smaller cities. Even in the South, which was less urbanized and where white men often seduced or raped black women, brothels began to appear in the cities. The mayor of Savannah, for example, estimated that there was one prostitute for every thirty-nine men in the city in 1858.[33]

In addition to the larger cities, prostitutes tended to also gather in areas where the ratio of men to women was high, such as the cattle and mining towns of the western territories. In the early years before the influx of families, most mining town residents, for example, were single men. In towns like Helena, Montana, and Comstock, Nevada, in the 1860s, the largest source of paid employment for women was prostitution. One scholar has estimated that prostitutes outnumbered other women in early mining towns by twenty-five to one.[34]

Venereal disease was seen more as a moral than as a medical problem at the time. Syphilis and gonorrhea were still often considered to be the wages of sin rather than a health problem to be tackled by community effort. In 1839, for example, Massachusetts General Hospital instituted a policy that venereally infected patients should only be received as "urgent cases" and should be charged double the usual rates. In New York City, nearly all of the venereal disease patients were treated at the Penitentiary Hospital on Blackwell's Island, the city's only facility for those so afflicted. In 1852, about 1,000 patients with venereal disease were admitted into this hospital. Many physicians refused to treat these diseases, opening the door to a host of quack doctors who offered confidential, quick "cures." There were also various patent medicines on the market that promised to cure these "secret" diseases. Some advertisements for cures even assured the patient that he could safely continue to have sexual relations with his spouse while undergoing treatment.[35]

As might be expected, the Civil War facilitated the expansion of prostitution and an increase in the incidence of venereal disease. Women interested in sexual commerce tended to gather wherever the men massed for training or battle. Union soldiers especially remarked upon the ready availability of prostitutes in the South. The social disruption caused by the war no doubt contributed to the situation. The poverty caused by the destruction of homes and farms pushed some southern women into prostitution. The number of brothels in the cities also increased during the war. For example, there were reportedly more than 400 brothels in Washington, DC. The slang term "hooker" for a prostitute derives from the fact that prostitutes "honored" General Joseph Hooker by naming the brothels around Lafayette Square in Washington "Hooker Row" (whether because he frequented the brothels or tried to limit them to this area is not known).[36]

Not surprisingly, venereal disease was not uncommon among the troops, although the incidence was substantially lower than that in most nineteenth-century European military forces. In all, there were a reported 73,382 cases of syphilis and 109,397 cases of gonorrhea and orchitis (an inflammation of the testes) treated in the Union army of about 600,000 men during the war. In other words, there were about 82 cases of venereal disease per 1,000 men. Although some writers have claimed that there was relatively little venereal disease in the Confederate army, H. H. Cunningham argues that it was more prevalent than generally supposed. For example, he cites the fact that there were forty-seven venereal admissions at Virginia's Emory Hospital from January, 1864 to April, 1865. Cunningham points out that only the cases with some complication that required hospital treatment got counted. Most cases were treated and kept in the field and never recorded. It is difficult to accurately estimate the actual incidence as most Confederate records were lost. After the war, many infected soldiers must have brought their diseases home to their wives and families.[37]

The incidence of venereal disease in the Union army varied significantly by region. For example, there was an epidemic of syphilis in the department of the Pacific (comprising the entire West Coast) in the first year of the war, with the number of cases reaching 218 by November, 1861. In general, the rate of venereal disease for the department of the Pacific for 1861–1862 was five times the national average for the Union army and represented one of the highest rates recorded for the United States military in the nineteenth century. The extent of venereal disease in the troops in New Mexico, although less than that in the Pacific region, was also higher than the national average. Murphy attributed the higher rate of venereal disease in the Far West to a higher proportion of men with attributes that made them more likely to engage in illicit sexual activity, military commanders who were less effective and conscientious in keeping the men away from prostitutes and insuring that the women were disease-free, and the level of venereal disease among the prostitutes.[38]

Prostitutes, who often doubled as laundresses, congregated near most military posts. Cincinnati, Chicago, Washington, Nashville, and Memphis were especially notorious for their numerous "bawdy houses." The concern about the threat to the health of soldiers by venereally infected women led to the first efforts at European-style regulation of prostitution in this country in the Union-occupied cities of Nashville and Memphis. In 1863, the Provost Marshal of Nashville instituted a system of legalized prostitution. Prostitutes would be licensed and subjected to weekly medical examinations. Infected women would be sent to a special hospital for treatment, with their care being financed by a fifty-cent weekly tax on each prostitute. Within a year of the initiation of the system, 456 white and 56 black prostitutes had registered. Military leaders felt that while this mechanism had not completely eliminated venereal disease, it had kept it under control.[39]

When Memphis was placed under martial law in July, 1864, the military officers in charge set up a system of licensed prostitution emulating that of Nashville. The Memphis system also involved regular medical inspection of the women, and "private female wards" were set up at the city hospital for the care of registered prostitutes (who could be treated for any disease free of charge). But legalized prostitution was not acceptable to most Americans, and the Nashville and Memphis systems were abandoned soon after the war ended.[40]

Mercury continued to be used in the treatment of syphilis, and, in desperation, military physicians tried a host of other methods as well. The chancres or ulcers of syphilis victims were sometimes cauterized (burned with a heated instrument or caustic substance). Steam baths were combined with mercury vapor. One doctor even tried using smallpox vaccination as a treatment for syphilis. Thomas Lowry wrote about the case of one poor soldier as follows:

> Surgeon E. A. Tomkins of Fort Yamhill, Oregon, described an unfortunate soldier with syphilis who, over a period of about four months, was treated with potassium iodide in sarsaparilla, corrosive sublimate, lunar caustic, calomel, black draught, emetics, blistering, iron, quinine, and external chloroform. At the end of the treatment, he was in severe pain, with one leg badly swollen and cold, barely able to walk.[41]

Venereal disease, of course, did not completely cease to be a problem in the military after the war ended. Soldiers and civilians stationed at military posts, especially in frontier areas such as the West, were generally separated from their families and frequently had relations with prostitutes who were attracted to these facilities. As Anne Butler has pointed out, no matter how isolated a fort was, the military did encounter local populations. In areas where the posts were near Indian populations, Indian women were sometimes employed as prostitutes, helping to spread the disease in these native populations. The 1887 report of the Commissioner of Indian Affairs cited 1,704 cases of venereal disease among Indians on all reservations. Butler also noted that part of the adaptation process of prostitution to both rural and urban frontier areas involved employment of available ethnic women (e.g., Mexicans, Asians, blacks, and Indians) as prostitutes.[42]

PHYSICIANS AND PROSTITUTES

As noted, the first attempts at the regulation of prostitution in the United States occurred under the military auspices of Union Army commanders in the occupied Southern cities of Nashville and Memphis, and did not long outlast the war. A few years after the end of hostilities, however, St. Louis became the first American city to experiment with the licensing of prostitutes by a civilian government. Following the Civil War, a number of American cities, including St. Louis, established boards of health, usually with a physician in charge. In 1870, Sr. William Barrett, the city's health officer, recommended that St. Louis institute a system of medical regulation of prostitution. Warning that prostitution was destroying the health of many inhabitants through venereal disease, and convinced that the practice could not be eliminated, he concluded that the best thing that could be done was to regulate it. Using a provision in the city charter to "regulate or suppress" prostitution, the City Council enacted the "Social Evil Ordinance" on July 5, 1870.[43]

The ordinance established a system of licensing and medical inspection of prostitutes. Six physicians appointed by the board of health, one in each of the city's six districts, inspected the registered women. Historian John Burnham further described the system as follows:

> Those women found afflicted with venereal disease were committed to a special Social Evil Hospital until certified cured. The Social Evil Hospital was to be financed by fees levied on licensed houses and individual prostitutes. Although amended several times, the Social Evil Ordinance remained in effect until 1874, when it was nullified by the Missouri state legislature.[44]

Although there was some disagreement among the members of the St. Louis Medical Society about the wisdom of the ordinance, the group did pass a resolution supporting it in 1871. The central thrust of their resolution, however, was a concern that some of the medical inspectors who had been appointed were not fully qualified. As John Duffy has pointed out, venereal disease was not a significant issue for discussion in medical journals until the passage of the St. Louis Ordinance. The St. Louis experiment, as Burnham noted, opened the door "to a national discussion of the hygienic value of government-enforced medical inspection of prostitutes."[45]

The increased interest of the medical profession in the regulation of prostitution and its relation to venereal disease in the period following the Civil War was part of a growing concern about public health. As epidemics of diseases such as cholera and yellow fever periodically affected the country, political and medical leaders recognized the need for a more organized approach to dealing with health issues. As previously mentioned, a number of cities began to establish local boards of health in this period. Several states had also established boards of health by the 1870s. Then, in 1872, a group of health reformers, including physicians and engineers, founded the American Public Health Association. At about this same time, the federal agency known as the Marine Hospital Service was beginning to expand beyond its mandate of providing medical care for merchant seamen to become involved with public health matters. The Quarantine Act of 1878, for example, conferred some quarantine authority on the Service for the first time.[46]

Although the St. Louis experiment ended in 1874, the debate over the regulation of prostitution continued. A number of prominent physicians were among the supporters of a system of licensing and inspecting prostitutes. In the very same year that the Missouri state legislature nullified the St. Louis ordinance, the eminent Philadelphia surgeon Samuel Gross, addressing the American Medical Association at its annual meeting in Detroit, argued the case for regulation. Expressing concern over the spread of venereal disease, Gross concluded that the only remedy for this problem was the licensing of prostitutes.[47] However, the membership of the Association disagreed on the issue of medical inspection of prostitutes, and did not approve Gross's request for an endorsement of the regulatory system.[48]

The question of regulation stirred up controversy in the medical establishment again in the 1880s. At the urging of Dr. Albert Gihon, Medical Director for the United States Navy, the American Public Health Association appointed a Committee on the Prevention of Venereal Diseases, with Gihon as chair, which was charged to pay special attention "to the protection of the innocent and helpless members of the community." The Committee, which claimed that it had tried to look at the issue in an unbiased way, presented its report at the Association's meeting in New Orleans in November 1880.[49]

The report emphasized the importance of educating the public to the fact that syphilis was not only the fruit of illicit sexual congress, but could lurk in even the most exemplary households. The disease is a serious problem that even affects "pure women and spotless children." The true incidence of venereal disease, according to the report, is unknown, since only a small percentage of cases are reported. The Committee did go on, however, to give what statistics they could find, namely data from hospitals and dispensaries for the poor in New York City and data from army, navy, and merchant marine hospitals from the 1870s. These various populations exhibited figures of from 44 to 225 cases of venereal disease for every thousand patients treated, with the numbers for syphilis running between 18 and 171 per thousand.[50]

The Committee voiced the opinion that if venereal diseases were restricted to those who sought illicit sexual gratification, "it might be well to let the guilty suffer and die." But there were also many "innocent victims" of venereal disease. A husband who had sex with an infected prostitute, for example, could bring the disease home to his wife. If she were pregnant, she could potentially pass it on to the unborn child. At the time, it was widely believed that syphilis could be contracted through a variety of types of contact. One suspects that physicians may even have exaggerated these beliefs, at least subconsciously, because they allowed victims of the disease to contend that they had not contracted it through sexual intercourse. The report maintains that syphilis could be communicated by kissing, from a public drinking vessel, from household articles such as towels or bed linens, and "through many thousand channels."[51] In dramatic fashion, the report highlights the dangers of syphilis:

> Every one instinctively shrinks from the touch of the sufferer with small-pox; but few realize that the syphilitic is a leper, also to be shunned! how few mothers are aware of the danger to themselves and their children from nurses and housemaids, drawn from a population in which every fifteenth person is diseased! how few parents suspect the peril to their daughter from her accepted lover's kiss, who may be that one in every five young men among the better classes, who has a venereal disease, which, there is one chance in two, is syphilis.[52]

What could be done about the scourge of venereal disease? The Committee provided statistics from various countries and from the Civil War experiment in Nashville, which, the report claimed, suggested that the licensing and medical inspection of prostitutes led to a decreased rate of venereal disease. The plan put forward in the report recommended a system of regulation of prostitution and the establishment of venereal disease hospitals or other methods of free treatment as an effective, practical means of preventing the spread of venereal disease. Brothels, the report admitted, are "monstrous blots upon the civilization of this century," but that was a matter of public morals rather than public health. The Committee emphasized, furthermore, that recommending the regulation of prostitution "no more implies the recognition and countenance of the sin of immorality than the license of rum-shops and the taxation of whiskey presuppose the encouragement of intoxication." Finally, the report recommended that the Association pass a resolution encouraging state and local boards of health to make it a criminal offence to knowingly communicate a contagious disease (including venereal diseases) to another.[53]

The report was published in 1881, and there was a lively discussion of the committee's recommendations at the following year's meeting of the American Public Health Association. John Shaw Billings, head of the Army Medical Library, moved to table the subject, commenting that even the discussion of it had caused religious groups to bring pressure to bear on the Association. Billings was concerned that endorsing the regulation of prostitution, by provoking opposition in many communities, would interfere with the ability of the Association to deal with broader public health concerns such as sanitation. The members present agreed with Billings by a thirty-eight-to-twenty vote. Although disappointed, Gihon said that he would not bring the matter up again to the Association, but he did not intend to entirely give up working on the problem.[54]

Aside from the concerns expressed by Billings, some physicians were opposed to regulation because they did not believe it was all that effective in combating venereal disease. They pointed out that there would no doubt be many prostitutes who would not register and therefore not be inspected, and also that the inspection process was not reliable. Before the introduction of the Wasserman test to diagnose syphilis in 1906, medical inspection was basically visual. Critics of regulation doubted the ability of physicians to detect syphilis by inspection in women. There was also nothing to prevent a woman from contracting a venereal disease in the interval between inspections.[55]

There were also reformers who wanted to abolish prostitution rather than regulate it. Unlike those who accepted prostitution as a necessary evil, a mechanism that provided an outlet for the sexual drive of men, these reformers believed that men could and should control their sexual urges. Middle class American women, in particular, were opposed to the double standard where men were given sexual license and women paid the penalties for illicit sex. Suffragists also opposed prostitution and sympathized with prostitutes as victim of men's lust. Many clergymen still saw prostitution in terms of sin, rather than as a public health matter. Reformers fought the efforts to establish a system of legalization and regulation of prostitution. D'Emilio and Freedman have noted that:

> When doctors recommended that Americans adopt regulated prostitution, they sparked a counteroffensive much larger than their own initial efforts toward regulation. The suggestion that the state should officially recognize prostitution as a necessary evil struck a sensitive chord among clergymen, former abolitionists, and women's rights activists. Together they organized formidable resistance to legalized prostitution. In Missouri, clergy and women succeeded in overturning the St. Louis experiment in 1874. Susan B. Anthony convened women's meetings to explain the implications for women's rights of the proposed New York legislation to regulate prostitution. Opponents of regulation helped defeat each of the New York State bills.[56]

The American efforts were part of a broader international reform movement. In 1877, an international congress was held in Geneva, Switzerland, for example, to promote abolition of what was called "State regulated vice." The meeting was attended by over 500 delegates from 15 countries. The congress participants challenged the ideas that prostitution was a necessity and that licensing of it reduced the incidence of venereal disease.[57] American reformer Aaron Powell, in reporting on the congress, also argued that legalized prostitution subordinated women and provided immunity to men. He wrote, "No woman ever does or can, as a prostitute, alone communicate syphilis to anybody. The guilty partner in her shame is always the special carrier and propagator of the disease."[58]

A NEW CENTURY DAWNS

As the nineteenth century drew to a close, the cause of syphilis was still unknown, and there was no definitive diagnostic test or effective treatment for the disease. That situation was shortly about to change. As discussed in the previous chapter, the first decade of the new century witnessed the isolation of the microorganism that caused syphilis, the introduction of the Wasserman test for diagnosing the disease, and the discovery of the drug Salvarsan for its treatment.

As historian Allan Brandt has demonstrated, concern over venereal disease increased substantially in early twentieth-century America for a variety of reasons, such as an increasing understanding of the long-term effects of syphilis in particular on the body. It was shown, for example, that syphilis could eventually lead to cardiovascular disease, partial or complete paralysis, and even insanity. Indirectly, through its devastating effects on the health of the individual, it could lead to pauperism and other social problems. Perhaps most influential according to Brandt, however, were fears about the negative impact of venereal disease on family life.

The growing tendency toward later marriages and smaller families coupled with an increase in the divorce rate caused Americans to worry about the demise of the middle-class family. By 1900, for example, the average American family had about 3.5 children, down from 6 in 1840. Especially troubling to many Americans was the fact that families of Anglo-Saxon stock were producing fewer children than the immigrants of "degenerate stock" from Eastern and Southern Europe, who had been flooding into the country since the late nineteenth century. Americans of Northern European ancestry feared that the descendents of immigrants such as Italians and Russian and Polish Jews would come to outnumber them.[59]

The early twentieth century was the heyday of eugenics in the United States. Born in England in the mind of Francis Galton, a cousin of Charles Darwin, eugenics billed itself as a science designed to produce a healthier human race by encouraging the reproduction of the "fit" and discouraging that of the "unfit." To many American eugenicists, that meant encouraging the reproduction of middle-class, white, Anglo-Saxons, as opposed to the newer immigrants and non-whites. Eugenicists also frequently advocated the sterilization of the mentally retarded, habitual criminals, sexual "perverts," and other "undesirables."[60]

Venereal disease, especially syphilis, fanned the flames of these fears in a number of ways. With respect to the decline of the family, reformers had already begun to point out in the nineteenth century that there were many "innocent victims" of venereal disease, as noted earlier. Wives who contracted the disease because their husbands had sex with infected prostitutes, or children born with congenital syphilis because the mother was infected, are examples of such innocents. Thus syphilis (as well as gonorrhea) came to be viewed as a "family poison."[61] Some physicians "came to view venereal disease as a threat to the very foundations of the Victorian, child-centered family; the susceptibility of innocent women and children seemed not only criminal, but treasonous."[62]

Syphilis and gonorrhea also figured in eugenic concerns. Physicians thought of syphilis as a hereditary disease, since it could be passed on from the mother to the newborn child, even though it is not necessarily the result of a genetic defect. Gonorrhea in the mother could also result in blindness in the newborn. Thus venereal diseases came to be thought of as causing degeneration of the race. One physician observed about syphilis, "No other disease is so susceptible of hereditary transmission, and so fatal to offspring." It was also believed that venereal infections contributed significantly to infertility in women, thus lowering the birth rate and contributing to what was called "race suicide."[63]

Venereal disease also entered into the debate about immigration. It was widely believed that arriving immigrants were frequently infected with these diseases. Although the Public Health Service physicians who examined the arrivals at Ellis Island found few cases of syphilis in the early years of the twentieth century, critics claimed that the examination for this disease was a "farce." Dr. Antonio Stella, an

Italian-born physician who emigrated to the United States, was still combating in the 1920s what he considered to be "wild accusations" that syphilis was commonly arriving with Italian immigrants. Stella pointed out that in July of 1921, over 11,000 immigrants were examined at Ellis Island and there were only 43 reported cases of venereal disease. It was also rumored that some immigrants, believing that sexual intercourse with a virgin could cure a venereal disease, were raping their own children. Many observers also believed that a majority of the prostitutes in American cities were foreign-born. Some claimed that thousands of immoral women as well as innocent girls were being imported into the United States every year as prostitutes.[64]

The connection of syphilis to racism with respect to African Americans also clearly emerged around the turn of the twentieth century. James Jones has pointed out that up until about 1890, American physicians discussed syphilis within the confines of what they considered to be the declining health of blacks in general. Although there were occasional remarks about the "sexual immorality" of blacks, this view did not form a theme. By the beginning of the new century, when race relations reached a low point, physicians became more critical of the lifestyle of African Americans. Although still believing that blacks were inherently more susceptible to disease than whites, physicians now began to place more blame directly on blacks for their perceived poor health. Blacks were chastised for ignoring personal and community hygiene, as if they were solely responsible for the socioeconomic conditions under which many poor blacks lived.[65] Jones went on to say:

> In this atmosphere it was not surprising that physicians depicted syphilis as the quintessential black disease. Most practitioners no doubt agreed with an instructor in neurology at Northwestern University who asserted that blacks contracted syphilis because of their "ever-increasing low standards of sexual morality."[66]

Many Americans believed that both black men and women had low moral standards, being completely lacking in virtue and chastity. There was a certain morbidity, as John Haller, Jr., stated, in the preoccupation of physicians with the sexual appetites of blacks. In addition to a belief in the excessive sexual passion of blacks, it had also long been widely accepted that they had sex organs that often reached massive proportions. The penis of the black male, for example, was reputed to be significantly larger than that of the average white male. African American men were sometimes depicted as being unable to control their sexual impulses. Many whites were also frightened by the myth that black men had a perversion that prompted them to attack Caucasian women.[67]

Physicians argued that because of this sexual indulgence, there was nothing to prevent the indiscriminate spread of syphilis among African Americans. Many white physicians despaired of being able to control the disease in the black community because they doubted that education could overcome the strength of the Negro's sexual drive. They also tended to believe that blacks did not take the disease seriously. One doctor described blacks as "a notoriously syphilis-soaked race."[68] Although there were no thorough and reliable statistics to back the claims that syphilis was much more common in blacks than whites, data from isolated studies were often cited as evidence confirming this general impression. Examples of statements from articles in medical journals in the first decade of the twentieth century that reveal the depth of these beliefs include the following:

> The negro springs from a southern race, and as such his sexual appetite is strong; all of his environments stimulate this appetite, and as a general rule his emotional type of religion certainly does not decrease it.[69]

> Both Quillan and Murrell state that they have never examined a negro girl over eighteenth years of age who was a virgin, and Hazen says the negro physicians of Washington admit that virginity is rare among the poorer members of the race. Herein lies the reason for the high ratio of syphilitics in the colored race, and until some curb is placed upon this promiscuous sexual communication in this class of these people, or until proper therapeutic measures are forced upon them, syphilis will run rife among them and threaten those of us with whom they come in contact.[70]

> It is my honest belief that another fifty years will find an unsyphilitic negro a freak, unless some such procedure as vaccination comes to the relief of the race, and that in the hands of a compelling law.[71]

Physicians and others were also concerned that the nation was undergoing an epidemic of venereal disease. The Committee of Seven appointed by the New York County Medical Society to assess the problem of venereal disease, for example, reported that between 5 and 18 percent of men suffered from syphilis. Estimates for the number of men who had been infected with gonorrhea at one time of another were even higher. Statistics from the Army in 1909 indicated that the admission rate for venereal disease was close to 200 per thousand. For the general population, however, venereal disease statistics continued to be unreliable. Given the social stigma associated with venereal infections, medical authorities were reluctant to report cases and compile statistics. Nevertheless, the medical profession was concerned that the rate of venereal disease was high and rising, although critics charged that moralists exaggerated these statistics in order to generate public concern.[72]

THE SOCIAL HYGIENE MOVEMENT

The early twentieth century is frequently referred to as the Progressive Era in America. Historical interpretations of Progressivism have changed over time, but it is not important for our purposes to delve into the subject in detail. It is sufficient to cite the brief summary given by D'Emilio and Freedman:

> A nationwide response by the middle class to the vast changes provoked by industrial capitalism, Progressive reform called upon the state to intervene as never before in the country's economic and social life. It addressed issues that ranged from the need for playgrounds and housing codes in urban slums to checking the power of monopolistic trusts. As a number of writers have pointed out, the Progressive movement embodied sharply conflicting impulses—social order as well as social justice, efficiency along with uplift, faith in the power of education as well as a determination to coerce the recalcitrant.[73]

Progressives, under President Theodore Roosevelt, undertook national efforts to break up large trusts, regulate railways, ensure pure foods and drugs, and enact various other political and economic reforms. As *The Oxford Companion to United States History* has noted, however, the Progressive movement was as much a cultural, and even a religious, phenomenon as a political one. The *Companion* commented, "Progressive leaders came from Protestant and often clerical families, they had learned Christian moral principles from an early age, and they tended to assume that sin was somehow at the core of social problems."[74]

Progressives were as concerned as many other middle-class Americans about the changes that immigration and industrialization were effecting on the nation, resulting in a more diverse culture. Nancy Bristow has noted that the Progressives, confident of the superiority of their own white, middle-class, urban habits and values, "set out to remake American culture" in their own image. Moralism was an important part of their agenda. Progressives tended to be especially concerned about the leisure patterns and morals of the working class. Men of the working class were often viewed by the reformers as sexually lascivious and uncontrolled. Working-class women were sometimes stereotyped as being ignorant and too ready to indulge in sex.[75]

As D'Emilio and Freedman have pointed out, issues of sexual morality easily fit within the Progressive framework. Some reformers preached education as the means to slow the spread of sexual vice and disease, while others called for repressive measures such as the eradication of prostitution. D'Emilio and Freedman went on to state:

> Of the many issues inviting attention, venereal disease was one that especially aroused reform energies... Despite the efforts of nineteenth-century social purity crusaders to address the problem, reticence about sexual matters still placed major obstacles in the way of forthright discussion of venereal disease. Although the improved social stature of the medical profession made it an ideal candidate for the job, any campaign against the diseases promised to clash with key elements of middle-class moral codes.[76]

This continued hesitancy to discuss sexual matters is reflected in the terminology used in newspapers and other public media of the early twentieth century. For example, the term "social evil" is consistently used in reference to prostitution, which is generally not mentioned by name. Similarly, syphilis and gonorrhea were referred to as "social diseases." And the effort to combat these problems was referred to as the "social hygiene" movement.

Prince Morrow, a New York physician, is generally regarded as the "Father of Social Hygiene." Morrow was born in Kentucky in 1846 and received his medical training in Europe. He began practicing medicine, in particular dermatology and syphilology, in New York in 1874, and eight years later he also received an appointment on the clinical faculty of New York University. In 1901, Morrow chaired the Committee of Seven of the New York County Medical Society on venereal disease mentioned earlier. It was apparently his attendance in 1902 as a United States delegate at the International Conference on Prophylaxis of Syphilis and Venereal Disease in Brussels, however, that stimulated him to become a crusader against venereal disease. Upon returning from this meeting, he immediately began to speak and write on the subject.

In 1904, Morrow published a book on *Social Disease and Marriage*, in which he emphasized the toll that syphilis and gonorrhea took on marriage and family life. He told of sterility among women, congenital blindness in infants, insanity, and other problems that these infections could introduce into the family. He spoke of the "innocent victims," the wives and unborn children, who might contract the disease because of the indiscretion of the husband and father. And he traced these infections ultimately back to prostitution. However, Morrow agreed with those nineteenth-century reformers who had placed the blame on the male client rather than the female prostitute.[77] He wrote:

> The male factor is *par excellence* the disseminator of venereal disease. He is chiefly responsible for its social consequences.... The prostitute is but the purveyor of the infection; she returns to one or several consumers the infection she has received from another consumer; her pathogenic activities are confined to the field of immorality; while in this field she is undoubtedly the more active spreader of contagion, she rarely invades the habitations of virtue. It is her partner who carries the infection home and distributes it to his wife and children.[78]

Morrow also opposed the "conspiracy of silence" on venereal disease, believing that ignorance and prudishness were responsible for the high incidence of syphilis and gonorrhea. He complained that social sentiment held that it was a greater impropriety to mention venereal disease publicly than to contract it privately.[79] The New York physician also argued that the public should be made fully aware of the consequences of contracting a venereal infection. In 1909, he wrote in a letter:

> Some of our educators maintain that our whole educational programme should be constructive in character and should touch little or not at all on the diseases which are practically inseparable from irregular living. On the contrary, I have always felt that the doctrine of consequences should be fully expounded, as the fear of infection will

sometimes restrain men from an evil life when educational or moral considerations will not avail. As a matter of fact, all hygienic precepts are based upon the consequences which result from the infraction of Nature's laws.[80]

Convinced that there was a need for an organization to deal with the problems of prostitution and venereal disease, Morrow formed the American Society for Sanitary and Moral Prophylaxis in 1905. The professed aim of the Society was to prevent the spread of diseases that had their origin in the "social evil." The organizational meeting at the New York Academy of Medicine was attended by twenty-five physicians. Believing that venereal disease was not strictly a medical issue, Morrow soon reached out to clergy, educators, journalists, and others to expand his organization, which grew to a membership of nearly 700 by 1910. In that same year, similar groups that had been founded in a number of cities, such as Philadelphia and Detroit, came together with Morrow's organization to establish the American Federation for Sex Hygiene under his leadership.[81]

At about this time, most large American cities also began to organize vice commissions to combat prostitution. These commissions emphasized that prostitution was a particular problem in cities. Young men looking for work migrated to urban areas, where they were away from the watchful eyes of family and neighbors and were often lonely. The cost of living was high and wages were low, and so young bachelors frequently postponed marriage. The cities also offered more opportunities for social contacts between the sexes, at dance halls, movie theaters, and other amusement venues. As more women entered the workplace, the vice commissions noted, social contacts between the sexes also increased. Some observers pointed out that women who had to earn their living sometimes turned to prostitution because it offered more lucrative earnings than many low-wage jobs. And single young women who lived separate from their families were subject to the same loneliness and temptations as young men in that position.[82]

There were also concerns in the early twentieth-century about so-called white slavery. Many vice crusaders were convinced that there was a ring of procurers operating in American cities to entrap young women and girls and force them into prostitution. The origin of the term "white slavery" has frequently been attributed to an Illinois assistant State's Attorney and crusader against involuntary prostitution. Supposedly he used the term at the beginning of the twentieth century when he was involved in a case in which a girl threw a note from a house of prostitution asking for help because she was being held captive as a "white slave." Historian of prostitution Vern Bullough, however, believes that the term more likely derives from an English translation of the French term "Traite de Blanches" (trade in whites), which was used at a 1902 international conference of European nations to discuss the issue of international traffic in women and children. It was probably used in distinction to the phrase "Traite des Noires" (trade in blacks), which had been employed in an earlier international conference on the black slave trade.[83]

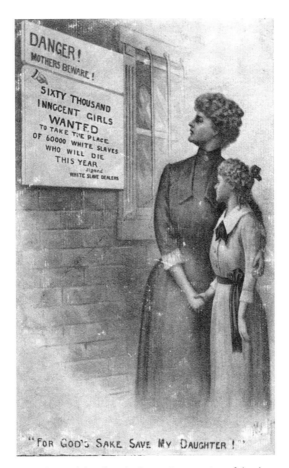

A mother and daughter look at a sign warning of the dangers of the "white slave" trade, a term used to refer to the practice of forcing women into prostitution. In the late nineteenth and early twentieth centuries, many believed that the practice of white slavery was widespread. From Clifford G. Roe, *The Great War on White Slavery* (1911).

Although enforced prostitution has existed since ancient times, American concerns seem to have first been aroused in the late nineteenth century by investigations of the "white slave trade" in Britain. There has been considerable historical debate about whether or to what extent the white slave trade existed in America in the Progressive Era. As historian Ruth Rosen has noted:

Whether increasing public concern about white slavery coincided with an actual increase in white slave traffic is difficult to determine. As a clandestine operation, the white slave trade obviously did not keep tidy historical records of its activities.[84]

The lack of records makes it impossible to quantify the level of white slave traffic in the United States in this period, but Rosen is convinced by the available evidence "that a trade in women, however small, existed." Certainly the belief in white slavery was widespread, and a subject of considerable concern. Beginning in 1908, several states adopted laws aimed at curbing white slavery, culminating in the passage by the federal government of the Mann Act in 1910. This law provided heavy penalties for the transporting or in any way aiding the transporting of women from one state to another for immoral purposes. Most states followed by enacting their own supplementary legislation against involuntary prostitution.[85]

While most social reformers agreed on a strategy of combating prostitution through education or through repression, there were still advocates of the view that prostitution would never be eliminated and that it was therefore best for the state to regulate it. Some physicians, in particular, continued to argue that licensing and inspecting prostitutes was the only sure means of controlling venereal disease. In 1910, the debate reached a climax when the State Legislature of New York passed the act popularly known as the Page Law. The act established a night court for women, required the fingerprinting of convicted prostitutes, and provided for the medical inspection of prostitutes. If a woman was found to be infected with a venereal disease, she could be detained for treatment. Opponents were outraged as they believed the law essentially established state-regulated prostitution. The New York Court of Appeals ended the debate over the law in 1911 when it found the section dealing with medical inspection and detention of prostitutes to be unconstitutional because it violated due process by making the diagnosis of the physician binding on the court.[86]

The battle over the Page Law seems to have served to unite the various social hygiene and antivice groups. Social hygienists tended to believe that sex education and public enlightenment were the best strategies for dealing with the problems of prostitution and venereal disease. They were especially concerned with the health aspects of the problem. The antivice organizations, on the other hand, focused more on white slavery and the repression of prostitution. Although Morrow recognized the advantages of combining forces, it was not until after his death on March 17, 1913 that these forces came together. Before his death, however, Morrow had persuaded a leading philanthropist to raise most of the funds needed to form a federation.

Several months after Morrow's death, leaders of his American Federation for Sex Hygiene and of the American Vigilance Association, an organization formed in 1912 that focused on eliminating the traffic in women, met in Buffalo to discuss a merger. The representatives voted to consolidate as the American Social Hygiene Association. John D. Rockefeller, Jr., who attended the Buffalo meeting, provided the greatest financial assistance to the new organization in its early years. In the previous year, Rockefeller himself had created a Bureau of Social Hygiene for the scientific study of prostitution and venereal disease. Charles W. Eliot, President Emeritus of Harvard University, agreed to serve as the first president of the American Social Hygiene

Association. Operation began on January 21, 1914, with the responsibility for management of the Association initially shared by James Bronson Reynolds, an attorney experienced in vice investigations, and physician William Freeman Snow, a professor at Stanford University and a California public health official. The Association's office was at first located in New York City.[87]

Snow, who soon became the Association's first executive director, discussed the origin and meaning of the phrase "social hygiene" in a 1916 report. He related that the term apparently originated in 1907 with the Chicago Society for Social Hygiene, a group that at the time was primarily concerned with sex education. He went on to define the term as follows: "Its present meaning is largely due to the necessity for some descriptive activities directed toward sex education, the reduction of venereal disease, and the repression of prostitution." Thus the new Association's name and its goals incorporated the concerns of the different groups of reformers which came together to found it.[88]

By the time of the Association's founding, a number of scientific breakthroughs in the first decade of the century had engendered new hope in the fight against syphilis. The isolation of the organism that caused syphilis, the development of a diagnostic blood test for the disease, and the discovery of a drug that seemed to offer effective treatment all occurred within the space of a few years. As Alan Brandt has explained:

> If syphilis could be properly diagnosed and effectively treated, as physicians now claimed, then it could be placed on the same footing by boards of health as other contagious diseases. Scientific advances opened the way for state and local public health officials to take a more aggressive stand in the fight against venereal diseases and to encourage the growth of the field of public health. In the period around the turn of the century, public health had been transformed from a broadly based movement dedicated to environmental reform to a more narrowly defined program emphasizing science, technique, and professionalism. As venereal disease came to be perceived as a scientific problem with a scientific solution, officials centered attention on communicable diseases and the bacteriological revolution that promised their demise.[89]

Brandt went on to point out that these developments resulted to some extent in a conflict between practicing physicians and public health officials. Many physicians were especially concerned that the privacy of their patients required them not to violate confidentiality in the case of venereal disease. Public health officials, on the other hand, argued that it was necessary for the control of infectious diseases that physicians report cases to the authorities. By this period, many cities and states required physicians to report cases of certain infectious diseases to boards of health so that officials could locate sources of infection, trace epidemics, and quarantine persons if necessary. Public health officials believed that venereal diseases should be included in such regulations. In 1911, under the leadership of William Snow, California became the first state to require physicians to report cases of venereal disease, although the reporting was done by number rather than name to protect the confidentiality of the patient. Other states and cities followed suit, but it appears that relatively few physicians complied with these regulations.[90]

Although an effective treatment could now be offered in the form of Salvarsan, facilities for treatment were inadequate. There were still prejudices against syphilis and gonorrhea in many hospitals. Doctors often argued against the establishment of out-patient clinics for diagnosing and treating venereal disease patients by boards of health because they believed that the state would be taking away patients from them. Brandt summed up the situation with respect to venereal disease at the time as follows:

> On the eve of the United States entry into World War I public health efforts against venereal disease remained haphazard. Physicians refused to pass their newly gained scientific and sexual authority to public health practitioners anxious to lead the fight against the disease. . . . Before World War I venereal disease, despite the remarkable scientific progress made in its diagnosis and treatment, was still distinguished from other infectious disease because it was sexually transmitted and thus evoked a certain moral repugnance. In fact, public health campaigns had come under attack for ignoring the moral aspects of the venereal problem. . . . Even physicians, nominally dedicated to scientific medicine, expressed concern that with the advent of effective therapy the value of venereal disease as a restraint against sexual license would be lost.[91]

THREE

"CONTINENCE IS NOT INCOMPATIBLE WITH HEALTH": SYPHILIS IN WORLD WAR I

PREPARATIONS FOR WAR

As it became increasingly evident that the United States was likely to be drawn into the conflict in Europe that erupted in 1914, the country began to make preparations. Expecting that America would enter the war, Congress established a Council of National Defense in August of 1916. Not surprisingly, given the experience of previous wars, concerns arose about the threat of venereal disease to the health of the American military. If it is true that Venus always accompanies Mars, i.e., that venereal disease and war are inextricably linked, then those preparing for America's entry into World War I were also preparing to fight syphilis and its ilk.

The American military had a "dress rehearsal" for the world war in the Mexican campaign that began with the incursion of Mexican rebel Francisco "Pancho" Villa into the southwestern United States in March of 1916. An army of 10,000 was sent to the area to deal with the invaders, and was primarily concentrated in towns along the Texas-Mexico border. Reports of immoral behavior among the troops soon began to reach military leaders and social reformers. In July, representatives of the American Social Hygiene Association (ASHA), the Rockefeller Foundation, and the Young Men's Christian Association (YMCA) met with Secretary of War Newton Baker to discuss their concerns about the moral situation on the front. As a result of the meeting, Raymond B. Fosdick, an investigator with Rockefeller's Bureau of Social Hygiene, was dispatched to Texas to observe the situation and report on it.[1]

Fosdick later recalled that he spent two months with the troops, making a survey of all camps on the Mexican border from Brownsville to the Gulf of California. He observed numerous houses of prostitution and saloons that catered to soldiers. While Fosdick was confident that these undesirable conditions could be eliminated, he came back with the feeling that no work of permanent value could be done without substituting something positive for what was being eliminated. He remembered standing in one camp and noting that there was nothing in the way of diversion of the troops—no books, magazines, canteens, or movies. He was convinced that part of the reason the men turned to saloons and prostitutes was because they were bored and had nothing else to do. These impressions had a lasting influence on Fosdick when he shortly thereafter was appointed head of a newly created agency to deal with conditions in and around military training camps.[2]

A representative of the YMCA, Max Exner, also surveyed conditions along the border. He also reported on the prevalence of saloons and prostitutes near the camps. Exner emphasized the problems that resulted from taking young men away from the normal restraining influences of home and family and putting them in an environment with temptations and opportunities for "debasement." Exner and Fosdick were both concerned with what they felt was the traditional military attitude that men required sex to be good soldiers. They believed that the army assumed that prostitution could not, and perhaps even should not, be eliminated. Many officers attempted to deal with the pervasive problem of venereal disease by having physicians inspect the local prostitutes on a regular basis.[3]

Given these conditions, it is not surprising that the rate of venereal disease in Texas was high. For troops in the San Antonio area, the rate was 288 per thousand. Secretary of War Baker did implement more strict disciplinary codes for soldiers and pressured local officials to "clean up" their communities, resulting in some improvement in conditions along the border. Baker did not at that time, however, implement Fosdick's recommendations about providing recreational activities for the soldiers.[4]

As Allan Brandt has noted, the implications of the border experience acquired new meaning as the prospect of American involvement in the world war increased.

> The problems of vice and disease on the Mexican border had been limited in both geo-graphical and numerical terms. The troops assembled there, moreover, had volunteered for service. A conscript army of American youth would entail greater federal responsi-bility. Entry into the war would transform the problem of sexually transmitted disease into a national issue of the first magnitude, requiring a centrally conceived program.[5]

On April 6, 1917, the United States entered the Great War and the military faced the prospect of housing large numbers of drafted men in training camps around the country. In the following months, President Wilson, the secretary of war, and the secretary of the navy received countless letters from citizens concerned about the moral well-being of the boys in uniform. Mothers and wives who accepted the necessity of their sons and husbands risking their lives in combat, for example, were not willing to tolerate their being ruined in body and ideals by immoral behavior. Citizens pleaded with their government to keep the soldiers "clean," free from the dangers of alcohol and illicit sex.[6]

Concerned that under the pressure of preparation for war, the issue of the moral environment of the training camps might not be addressed, Max Exner had published an article describing the conditions he had observed on the Mexican border. As he noted, "This article created much public discussion and stirred up all sorts of agencies and individuals to bring pressure to bear at Washington." Meanwhile, Fosdick developed a detailed proposal for a commission to oversee social and recreational activities in the training camps, as well as to control alcohol, prostitution, and other vices around the camps.[7]

The War Department moved quickly on April 17, 1917 to establish an agency along the lines recommended by Fosdick, the Commission on Training Camp Activities (CTCA). The Commission was charged with overseeing life within and immediately outside of the Army's training camps, with the goal of preventing the "moral decay" of the soldiers. Not surprisingly, Secretary of War Baker appointed Raymond Fosdick to serve as chairman of the CTCA. The Commission was designed to coordinate the activities of existing civilian organizations and to fill any identifiable gaps in the program itself.[8]

Other actions were also soon taken to help deal with the problem of vice in and around the training camps. The Selective Conscription Act, for example, was modified to prohibit the sale of alcoholic beverages to soldiers and to empower the secretary of war to do everything deemed necessary to prevent prostitution around military facilities. The leaders of the ASHA were also commissioned as military officers and asked to develop a program for the control of prostitution.[9]

Secretary of the Navy Josephus Daniels was also concerned about the moral health of the armed forces, arguing that nothing must be left undone in the effort to protect the men from "contamination" that would affect their military efficiency and their lives for the future. The title of a lecture that he delivered to a medical meeting was: "Men Must Live Straight If They Would Shoot Straight." Secretary Daniels was interested in putting a plan similar to the CTCA into operation for the Navy. In the minutes of its meeting of June 28, 1917, the CTCA reported that the Navy was setting up its own commission, and that some members of the CTCA might be asked to serve on it.[10]

The Council of National Defense likewise established a Committee for Civilian Cooperation in Combating Venereal Diseases (CCCCVD) to assist in controlling venereal disease in the civilian population. The national body worked closely with the various state Councils of Defense that had been established. Already on May 26, 1917,

Secretary Baker, using the letterhead of the Council of National Defense, wrote to the state Councils soliciting their assistance. He emphasized that the military would not be able to maintain the health and vitality of its soldiers without the full cooperation of local authorities in the areas near where the training camps would be located or through which the soldiers would pass in transit. He urged the state Councils to impress upon local officials their responsibility for "clean conditions" (with regard to saloons and prostitutes), which he considered a "patriotic opportunity."[11]

In a 1918 letter to a member of the United States House of Representatives, the executive secretary of the Council of National Defense voiced even more strongly the need for civilian cooperation in controlling venereal disease in the military. He wrote:

> Although the problem of venereal diseases in the Army and Navy is one of the most serious of all military problems, the War and Navy Departments are helpless without the cooperation of civil communities. During recent mobilizations a large amount of venereal disease has been brought from civil life into the Army and virtually all venereal disease in the Army and Navy originates in civil life.[12]

The overall wartime plan for protecting soldiers from venereal disease, involving these agencies and others, stressed legal repression of prostitution, prompt medical treatment for infected soldiers, provision of "wholesome" recreational opportunities in and near training camps, and venereal disease education for recruits. The program was designated the "American Plan." By contrast, the European military placed greater emphasis on the prevention and control of venereal disease through medical measures rather than through education in sexual hygiene and repression of prostitution.[13]

The American Plan rejected the idea, especially common in the military, that vice, and especially sexual activity, was inevitable wherever armies gathered. Social hygienists and reformers, in the words of Allan Brandt, "refused to accept the notion that American entry in the war would be accompanied by a dissipation in sexual morals and an increase in venereal disease."[14] They disputed claims about the uncontrollable nature of the male's sexual drive and about the harmful effects of suppressing sexual desires and activity. Medical professionals reassured the military that sexual abstinence would not harm soldiers. The Medical Board of the Council of National Defense declared that "continence is not incompatible with health and is the best preventive of venereal disease" and an official army bulletin stated that "[s]exual intercourse is not necessary for good health, and complete continence is wholly possible."[15]

In addition to protecting soldiers in training and transit on the home front, military leaders of course recognized that when American troops arrived in Europe they would be exposed to the threat of venereal disease there, and the leadership took precautions to attempt to minimize this risk. However, the venereal disease rate in the American Expeditionary Forces (AEF) was actually quite low, 3.4 percent, as

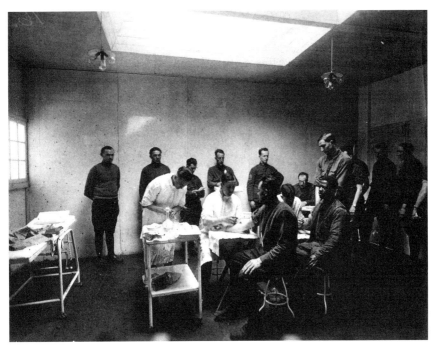

Men receiving Salvarsan treatment for syphilis at a United States Army base hospital in Nantes, France, World War I [Courtesy of the National Library of Medicine].

opposed to 12.7 percent of the men stationed within the United States. Although the Army Medical Department emphasized the importance of the role of educating the troops to avoid sexual contacts, other factors no doubt also played a role in the low infection rate. One official, for example, estimated that chemical prophylaxis had reduced the venereal disease rate to about one-third of what it would otherwise have been. Soldiers who had been exposed to venereal disease were required to receive chemical prophylaxis, which involved the injection of a chemical solution into the penis as well as external treatment of the penis with an ointment. These procedures were believed to greatly reduce the risk of venereal disease, although statistics showed that 55 percent of the soldiers who contracted a venereal disease had undergone the treatment. Soldiers who contracted a venereal disease and had not taken prophylaxis were subject to additional penalties. Brandt has also suggested other factors that may have contributed to the comparatively low venereal disease rate in the AEF, such as the strict provisions for discipline and prophylaxis in France and the French inspection of prostitutes.[16] The interested reader will find a more detailed discussion of this subject in George Walker's *Venereal Disease in the American Expeditionary Forces* and in Brandt's book.[17]

THE COMMISSION ON TRAINING CAMP ACTIVITIES

The CTCA took a leading role in protecting American soldiers on the home front from venereal disease. Fosdick indicated that there would be two sides to the work of the Commission, a negative or police side and a positive or creative side. He also made it clear that the Commission would not create any more "machinery" than was necessary, but would instead work with the aid of existing organizations as much as possible.[18]

In a booklet describing the work of the Commission, the War Department pointed out that the young men in the training camps have left behind all the normal social relationships (e.g., family, friends, churches) to which they have been accustomed and have entered a strange new life. The task of the Commission was "to re-establish, as far as possible, the old social ties" by furnishing the men with "a substitute for the recreational and relaxational opportunities to which they have been accustomed." The Commission was also tasked with the prevention and suppression of "certain vicious conditions traditionally associated with armies and training camps."[19]

The booklet went on to explain that the Commission had utilized the services of various existing organizations and agencies, rather than creating new machinery, in its work. For example, the YMCA and the Knights of Columbus provided a large share of the club life and entertainment in the camps. The American Library Association was providing books and reading facilities. The Playground and Recreation Association of America, along with other groups such as the YMCA, worked with local groups such as clubs and churches to organize social and recreational activities in the communities surrounding the camps. In dealing with the vice conditions around the camps, the CTCA cooperated with the ASHA, local police organizations, and other groups.[20]

When the first major draft of the war occurred in the fall of 1917, health and military officials realized that the venereal disease problem among the recruits was even more serious than they had anticipated. As historian Edward Beardsley has explained:

> By the end of the second week of mobilization, the [venereal] disease rate for the new conscript army had vaulted to 357 cases per 1000 men, about four times the Regular Army rate, while in the National Guard it had climbed to 150. In the period from September 1917 until the following May, some 80,000 cases were discovered among the new soldiers, most of whom brought their infection into the army from civilian life.[21]

Understandably, the military was concerned about having further numbers of men infected while they were in training. The CTCA thus implemented a variety of programs to occupy the time of the men and to keep them away from liquor and prostitutes. The more optimistic of the reformers saw an opportunity not only to keep the soldiers healthy, but to morally uplift them. The CTCA itself saw its work proceeding along four lines: (1) provision of amusement and recreational resources (e.g., movies, game rooms) in the camps; (2) organization of athletic activities within the camps; (3) mobilization of recreational and social agencies in communities near the camps to provide opportunities for wholesome recreation and social life for men on leave; and (4) regulation, inspection, and control of public amusements in the neighborhoods of the camps.[22] The CTCA eventually consisted of three major divisions: Intracantonment Recreation (responsible for recreational activities within the training camps), Extracantonment Recreation (responsible for recreational activities in the communities surrounding the camps), and Prevention of Venereal Disease (responsible for protecting the servicemen against venereal infections).[23]

PROSTITUTION AND KHAKI FEVER

The military placed substantial pressure on local communities where camps were established, or soon would be, to clean up their act. An important first step in the mind of military and civilian leaders was the elimination of red-light districts in the areas around the training camps. In a letter dated August 10, 1917 to leaders in communities where training camps were soon to open, for example, Secretary Baker provided a copy of the recently established regulations on the suppression of prostitution and the sale of alcohol to soldiers in uniform within a given radius of the camp. He went on to explain that while the War Department had set this radius at five miles for prostitution, it would not tolerate "evil resorts of any kind within easy reach of the camp." Baker emphasized that this policy required constant vigilance on the part of the police, involving not only eliminating houses of prostitution, but also "checking the more or less clandestine class that walks the streets and is apt to frequent lodging houses and hotels." He asked for the cooperation of local officials and alerted them that the CTCA would be advising him on these matters and reporting to him on conditions around the camps.[24]

Bascom Johnson, counsel to the ASHA, was in charge of the CTCA's efforts to eliminate prostitution and alcohol in the cities near the training camps. He received the rank of Major in the Army Sanitary Corps. Vice investigators went to various regions of the country to inspect and report on local conditions in cities near the camps. They worked with local officials and citizens to close down red-light districts and otherwise "clean up" the communities. The military was not averse to applying pressure to achieve these goals. For example, Raymond Fosdick wrote to the Attorney General of Alabama on July 7, 1917 to inform him that the secretary of war had asked him to say that "the War Department cannot tolerate in the vicinity of a training camp a restricted district for public women" and that "if such districts are not effectively abolished, and the prostitutes removed, the Secretary is determined to change the location of the camp." By the fall of 1917, the CTCA had succeeded in having many red-light districts closed. This did not end the problem, however, as prostitutes just resorted to using hotels, rooming houses, dance halls, and other venues to ply their trade. Street walkers also became more common. Venereal disease rates in the camps remained high.[25]

Reports from Bascom Johnson on his travels in California in July of 1917 illustrate the investigations of the "moral conditions" surrounding military camps. Johnson reported that the red light district of San Francisco had been closed as early as February of that year, but that there were still hundreds of prostitutes operating in the city, especially in the Barbary Coast dance halls and the "uptown tenderloins." Some of the hotels were notorious for serving as places where prostitutes could entertain their clients. In San Diego, Johnson and his colleagues found prostitutes soliciting business in cafes, hotel dining rooms and bars, and on the streets. The night porter at the hotel where Johnson was staying, a "better class moderate priced" facility, even offered to send a woman to his room. The closeness to Tia Juana, Mexico, "always an open town for prostitution," also created problems for San Diego because of "the procession of disreputable characters to and from its borders."[26]

By 1918, the CTCA had concluded that closing the red light districts had only shifted prostitution to more clandestine forms. As law enforcement cracked down on each type of prostitution, prostitutes turned to less easily detected methods of solicitation. Frustrated by the difficulty of eliminating the practice, the CTCA adopted a new strategy. As Nancy Bristow explained:

> Recognizing the flexibility and the resilience of prostitution as an institution, the CTCA concluded that ultimately prostitutes themselves, rather than the institution of prostitution, had to become the target of repressive efforts if the CTCA's antivice campaign was ever to succeed.[27]

The CTCA decided that in order to eliminate prostitutes, they would need a system of detention houses and reformatories to detain these women. By this time, the CTCA had come to a similar conclusion with respect to women who were not actually prostitutes, but who were considered to be promiscuous by the CTCA and its allies. From its founding, the CTCA believed that the health and moral well-being of soldiers could be undermined by promiscuous women and girls as well as by prostitutes. They could spread venereal disease to the troops as easily as prostitutes could. One group that concerned the CTCA was seemingly innocent young girls who had caught "khaki fever" (i.e., lost control at the sight of a uniform), a stereotypical view of women who were overcome by their feelings. More mature women who had always been "free" with their sexual favors also worried the CTCA.[28]

The concern with the "girl problem" did not begin with the war. American reformers had been concerned about the sexuality of young women, especially working class women, since at least the late nineteenth century, when working class women began to rebel against the constraints of Victorian morality. Young working women, often living apart from their families, had more freedom to socialize with men. Dance halls, movies, and amusement parks provided opportunities for socializing in the dawn of the twentieth century. A subculture of working women traded sexual favors in exchange for being treated to an evening out or for gifts. In underworld slang, these women were referred to as "charity girls," to distinguish them from prostitutes, because they did not accept money for sex.[29]

The attention paid to "charity girls" by reformers naturally increased during the war, and the use of the term broadened. As described by Bristow:

> During the war the term took on additional meaning. Although it might still refer to women using sex as part of an exchange relationship, it also came to refer to any woman who engaged in sexual relations with soldiers free of charge.[30]

When the CTCA was first established, there was an effort to try to distinguish between these women and prostitutes. A Committee on Protective Work for Girls (CPWG) was created in September of 1917. The strategy was to protect "khaki-crazed" girls from the dangers of predatory men or from their own "foolish" choices, and to prevent women from becoming prostitutes in the first place (since Fosdick saw this as the inevitable next step for promiscuous women). Maude Miner, secretary of the New York Probation and Protective Society, became the first chairwoman of the CPWG. Miner and her staff tried to emphasize the protective and constructive aspects of their work over the repressive ones. Protective workers patrolled the areas and communities near the training camps and befriended the girls that they found, warning them of their danger and referring them to other organizations when appropriate. They tried to persuade the girls not to act foolishly and unwisely.

In spite of the attempt to emphasize the positive, there was a repressive side to the activities of the CPWG as well. When protective workers found girls violating the law, they were supposed to take them into custody or to notify the authorities so that the girls could be detained. However, the workers were expected to use police powers only when necessary. The CPWG also encouraged its local branches to work for the creation of detention homes in their communities, so that the girls would not have to be housed in jails with experienced prostitutes and hardened criminals.[31]

Over time, the CTCA increasingly emphasized repression over protection. Miner and her coworkers found that their assumptions that the girls they targeted were simply misguided, without proper supervision, and victims of predatory men were not always true. Miner had assumed that the girls could easily be encouraged to adopt middle-class values and "proper" standards of behavior. As the work progressed, however, she began to realize that many of the girls consciously rejected middle-class standards and chose to be sexually active. Although she came to recognize the need for more detention homes to house recalcitrant girls, she believed that the CPWG should retain control of the reformatory work and she continued to emphasize a protective approach. Fosdick, who was naturally focused on the protection of soldiers against venereal disease, disagreed with Miner, arguing that the priority of the CTCA should be to incarcerate girls who posed a risk to soldiers.[32]

As described by Linda Janke, CTCA policy toward these women changed over time:

> As CTCA officials' impression of delinquent women and girls evolved, CTCA staff adjusted their approach. Rather than seeking to protect endangered girls, CTCA leaders began to emphasize protecting soldiers. In light of these altered priorities, Fosdick decided to reorganize the CTCA's work for girls. In early 1918, he opted to discontinue Miner's plan to intervene on an individual level with each potentially delinquent girl. Instead, CTCA policies emphasized a law enforcement approach designed to remove delinquent girls from the soldiers' presence. This reorganization entailed increased surveillance of working-class women and girls, mass arrests, venereal disease testing, and sentencing large numbers of women and girls to reformatories.[33]

As part of this reorganization, Fosdick created an entirely new unit within the Law Enforcement Division, the Committee on Reformatories and Detention Homes (CRDH), to handle the reformatory work. He hired Martha Falconer, a member of the CPWG with experience in juvenile justice, to head the CRDH. Falconer, as opposed to Miner, agreed with Fosdick that incarceration of delinquent girls was the best solution for protecting the nation's military strength. The CPWG was also replaced by a Section on Protective Work for Girls, which soon changed its name to the Section on Women and Girls (SWG), perhaps, as suggested by Nancy Bristow, because it did so little protective work. The new section combined the work with delinquent and charity girls with that for professional prostitutes. Unhappy with these changes, Miner resigned in April of 1918.[34]

The staff of the SWG viewed their work primarily as a law enforcement matter. A significant amount of their time was devoted to the problem of venereal disease, and they assisted the Law Enforcement Division (of which they were a part) in the incarceration of venereally diseased women. Rather than following the case-work approach of the CPWG, the SWG emphasized surveillance of girls who were likely to break the law. They concentrated on women who were already sex offenders and who were causing problems near the camps. In their words of Janke, "their protective work had changed: they now protected soldiers from delinquent girls."[35]

Incarcerating larger numbers of women required more facilities for this purpose. In February 1918, President Wilson allocated $250,000 for the purpose of establishing detention homes for women convicted of sex offenses. This funding allowed for the construction of eighteen new reformatories and the improvement of four existing ones. Then in July Congress enacted the Chamberlain-Kahn Bill, which included one million dollars for a "civilian quarantine and isolation fund." This money was to be used for the establishment of reformatories for the isolation and detention of civilians as necessary to protect the troops against venereal disease. However, the Comptroller of the Treasury ruled that the Interdepartmental Social Hygiene Board, the agency set up to administer the program, had no power to spend federal funds on construction or repair of facilities not owned by the federal government. Instead the funds were used to provide for the maintenance and treatment of women already in the custody of existing institutions. Less than one-fifth of the appropriation was actually spent. Allan Brandt has speculated that if the full one million dollars could have been used for a massive construction program of new facilities, many more women would have been quarantined under the program. As it is, more than 18,000 women, of whom 15,520 reportedly had a venereal disease, were committed to institutions receiving federal funding in the period between 1918 and 1920. These women were held on average for about ten weeks.[36]

Overall, some historians have estimated that as many as 30,000 women were incarcerated under the wartime programs. Others think that this figure might be an underestimate and that the actual number might be much higher. Since many women were incarcerated without documentation, it is difficult to be sure of the exact number. These incarcerations were carried out without a trial or legal due process.[37]

Many state and local governments, with the encouragement of the CTCA, passed laws requiring medical examination of citizens "reasonably suspected" of being venereally infected. A Virginia ordinance, for example, authorized health officers to examine vagrants, prostitutes, "persons not of good fame," and others who might reasonably be suspected of having syphilis or gonorrhea. No one arrested under this law could be released on bail until examined and found to be free of venereal disease. Thirty-two states had passed laws requiring compulsory examination of prostitutes for venereal disease by March 1918. The federal Department of Justice supported the practice of compulsory examination of arrested women, and courts tended to uphold quarantine rulings.[38] David Pivar has summarized the situation as follows:

> Enforcement officers arrested women suspected of prostitution and health boards conducted hearings. Writs of habeas corpus could be suspended. Women could be subjected to compulsory, inconclusive and painful examinations. If diseased, suspects could be sent to detention centers under indeterminate sentencing. According to the law, they would receive treatment for diseases and given vocational training.[39]

Treatment for syphilis involved injections of the new arsenical drug, Salvarsan, and often mercurial ointments as well, and was sometimes administered against the will of the patient. One pharmacology textbook of the period described a typical treatment regimen as involving three doses of Salvarsan (or the more soluble related compound Neosalvarsan), generally administered by intravenous injection, given over a period of several weeks, followed by treatment with mercury. The author noted that this course of therapy might have to be repeated at intervals until a permanent cure was effected. He also pointed out that the drug was less effective in the later stages of syphilis.[40] Some reformers, including a number of physicians, seemed relieved that Salvarsan was not an easy and sure cure for syphilis, believing that venereal disease played an important role in sexual morality by preventing people from sinning with impunity.[41]

In some of the institutions for the detention of women, treatment could be quite aggressive. For example, Nancy Rockafellar described the situation at a Seattle facility:

> Intravenous Salvarsan treatments were administered on a separate floor, often by force. Treatment regimens for syphilis were aggressive. Some women received as many as nineteen shots of Salvarsan, rubbed mercury until saturated.[42]

In 2007, Michael Lowenthal published the novel *Charity Girl*, based on the World War I program for the incarceration of women. In an explanatory note, Lowenthal stated that because it was difficult to distinguish "the criminal from the merely adventuresome," women were arrested for such "offenses" as dressing provocatively or being in certain neighborhoods without an escort. His fictional tale tells the story of Frieda Mintz, a young working girl in Boston who impulsively has sex with a soldier. She contracts a venereal disease and travels to the area of the army camp where the soldier is located in an effort to contact him. However, Frieda "is tracked down and sent to a makeshift detention center, where she suffers invasive physical exams, the discipline of an overbearing matron, and a painful erosion of self-worth." The novel paints a vivid picture of life at a detention center.[43]

After the war, Mary Macey Dietzler published a detailed report on the detention houses and reformatories that received federal support. Since army camps were concentrated in the South, a majority of the detention facilities were also located in this part of the country. The institutions varied greatly in their capacity, housing, opportunities for education or vocational training, supervised work time, recreational facilities, discipline, security, and medical care.[44] Some of the institutions more severely restricted the movement of inmates than others. Dietzler reported, not surprisingly, that the number of escapes was higher in facilities that allowed more freedom. The government reported, however, that nearly 90 percent of the patients remained institutionalized until they had been declared noninfectious.[45]

In addition to providing statistics and general information, Dietzler included a brief history of each of the individual institutions. Though there is no one institution that could be considered typical, the detention hospital in Montgomery, Alabama, can be considered as one example. The hospital consisted of two one-story frame cottages, one for white women and one for black women. Each cottage could hold twenty inmates. The facility was surrounded by a high barbed-wire fence. Patients were admitted under quarantine for the period of their infectivity. Female visitors were allowed, but fathers of the inmates were the only male visitors permitted to visit. The inmates were responsible for housekeeping and laundry, and also made their own garments. There was no formal instruction in music, but the women sang and danced a lot in the evening. Apparently there was not much else in the way of recreation. The inmates were treated for venereal disease by visiting physicians and nurses. The average length of stay of the patients was twelve weeks. Over the course of time, eighteen inmates escaped from the institution.[46]

The experience of World War I followed the age-old pattern of placing the major burden for the spread of venereal disease on women. A Public Health Service officer, for example, claimed that about 90 percent of infections were due to women. Men, he believed, took more precautions and were more inclined to seek treatment, whereas women were more negligent about such matters, although he offered no sound evidence for such claims.[47] Prostitutes and promiscuous women were sometimes compared to enemy bullets or spies, just as damaging in their effects on soldiers and national security.[48] They were scapegoats of the war. Edward Beardsley has commented that American reformers of the period, "seeking an outlet for a heightened nationalism, but not having any real live Germans and Austrians to confront, . . . focused on prostitutes and venereal disease as suitable substitutes."[49] One government official referred to the prostitute as committing "moral and social murder."[50] As Sarah Judson has noted:

> With her seductive wiles and her diseased body, the urban woman's sexuality was viewed as an instrument of treason, threatening not only the success of the U.S. army, but also the social and physical fabric of the American home. Similar to the menace of the German Kaiser, women who engaged in sex outside of marriage threatened the downfall of civilization.[51]

Any sexually active unmarried women was seen as a potential source of venereal disease, and often treated as a prostitute. It was also assumed that essentially all prostitutes were venereally infected, and that those who were not would soon be. Police and judges frequently took it for granted that any woman exhibiting "immoral behavior" was acting like a prostitute and hence most likely diseased. They often implicitly assumed that the disease was always transmitted from prostitute to customer, without considering how the prostitute contracted the disease in the first place.[52] One government educational pamphlet urged men to keep away from any kind of women willing to give them a "good time," whether for money or not, because 70 to 95 percent of prostitutes and "chippies" have syphilis or gonorrhea. Another government poster claimed that 70 percent of all "loose women" had both syphilis and gonorrhea. It is not known how these statistics, which seem highly suspect, were compiled.[53]

Clearly the wartime vice programs discriminated against women and reinforced the double standard for sexual activity. Women were generally punished by officials and the courts far more severely than men for sex offenses. When soldiers were caught having illicit sex with women, the soldiers were generally allowed to go free while the women were arrested. Soldiers in these situations might have been required to undergo chemical prophylaxis against venereal disease, but they were not arrested and incarcerated. Even civilian men were rarely treated in a way comparable to women. For example, although technically the state quarantine law in Texas included both men and women, it was not generally applied to men. There were no detention facilities built for the large-scale incarceration of men who had committed sexual offenses and/or were found to suffer from a venereal disease, although some men were held in detention during the war.[54]

The war provided a rationale for the need for apprehension and detention of women who posed a danger to soldiers in terms of venereal disease. Certainly, wartime fears and patriotism made these repressive measures more acceptable to many Americans. As a number of historians have pointed out, however, the campaign against these women went beyond battling venereal disease and prostitution. Middle-class reformers were troubled by young women, usually of the working class, who transgressed what they considered to be proper standards of behavior. They felt threatened by changing mores of female sexuality and considered these women to be delinquents.[55]

There were of course opponents who protested this discriminatory treatment of women, but they were in the minority. Dr. Katherine Bushnell, physician, Christian missionary and reformer, criticized the compulsory examination of women for venereal disease, comparing it to indecent assault. One California official complained that Bushnell had issued pamphlets opposing proposed Board of Health regulations in Oakland, claming that they were a revival of European contagious disease acts that discriminated against women. Chicago reformer Ethel Drummer was another vocal critic. Although Drummer worked for the CTCA, she was critical of the CTCA's policies toward women. She especially decried the double standard that incarcerated women but not men.[56]

RECREATION AND EDUCATION

Although limiting the access of soldiers to prostitutes, "loose women," and liquor was a key element of the CTCA's antivenereal disease campaign, it was not the only weapon in its arsenal. Fosdick believed that it was not enough to remove temptations from the path of the soldier; one needed also to provide healthy outlets to occupy his time. In addition, soldiers and civilians needed to be educated in the area of social hygiene, to emphasize the dangers of venereal diseases and to instill good moral standards.

With respect to recreation in and around the training camps, the CTCA relied to a significant extent upon existing organizations and institutions to implement these programs. The YMCA established "huts" in all of the camps where soldiers could write letters, listen to music, attend lectures and church services, and engage in other activities. The Knights of Columbus and the Jewish Welfare Board sponsored similar activities. The YMCA also established houses where wives and girlfriends could visit soldiers under chaperoned conditions. Athletic programs were also established, including football, basketball, and baseball games. Group singing was popular. The American Library Association established libraries in the camps.[57]

The YMCA and other groups brought amateur vaudeville entertainment and movies to the camps, but the CTCA was also interested in finding a way to provide the troops with regular programs of professional entertainment. The Regular Army Act of June 15, 1917 included $500,000 for the purpose of construction of theaters in the camps. Eventually these Liberty Theatres, ranging in size from about 1,000 to nearly 3,000 seats, were built in forty-three camps. Plays, motion pictures, and variety acts were featured in the theaters. Although the theaters were filled to only about one-third of their capacity on average for each performance, this was in part because they were really too large for the populations they were intended to serve. Overall, the theatres drew over 8.5 million patrons between January 1918 and August 1919, and earned $2.4 million in revenues (admission was charged) for the War Department. The revenues more than covered operating and talent expenses, leaving the War Department with a profit of about $270,000 that was used to subsidize entertainment in army facilities after September 1, 1919.[58]

The CTCA and its community counterpart, the War Camp Community Services (WCCS), also cooperated with communities near the training camps to develop recreation programs for soldiers. Some of these communities built swimming pools, comfort stations, and soldier clubs. Local churches and organizations sponsored dances, picnics, parades, concerts, and other activities for the servicemen. Families often invited soldiers home for dinner. Social activities where soldiers interacted with young women were supervised by the WCCS to ensure that they were carried out in the "proper" way. Beach parties, for example, were held only on moonlit nights or with sufficient light from lanterns and fires. The WCCS supervised dances by providing chaperones, and also regulated dress, lighting, music, and dance styles.[59]

The CTCA also established a social hygiene program that was responsible for venereal disease education for both soldiers and civilians. Initially, the focus of the Social Hygiene Instruction Division was on education in the Army camps (and later Naval facilities as well). Dr. Walter Clarke of the ASHA directed the Division. He drew upon proven advertising techniques to help persuade the soldiers to exercise sexual self-restraint, noting that the "selling" of conduct was similar to the selling of shoes or automobiles. The unit used posters, pamphlets, exhibits, lectures, etc. in the education of the troops. The CTCA preferred to stress rationality and science over moralism in these educational methods, fearing that the latter approach might alienate the soldiers. Emphasis was placed on the importance of soldiers staying healthy and fit to fight for the success of the war effort. However, sexual continence, a theme acceptable from both a medical and a moral point of view, became the basis of the educational efforts, and moral issues were not totally ignored.[60]

Although outside organizations such as the YMCA could distribute printed materials or offer lectures on sex education, these had to be approved by the CTCA and the Army Surgeon General. Lecturers had to be accredited by the CTCA. The Army also assigned military men to provide social hygiene instruction. At one point a noncommissioned officer was assigned to each camp to provide lectures on social hygiene.[61]

The Navy instituted a similar social hygiene instruction program, and the syllabus for use in the lectures on sex hygiene and venereal disease is essentially identical for both the Army and the Navy. The syllabus emphasizes that lecturers must avoid or explain technical and medical terms, using a simplified language that the troops could understand. Lecturers were told not to use words that, "while good in themselves," might "have unfortunately acquired prejudice in the minds of many men whom it is particularly desired to influence." This included all words with a theological or semi-theological connotation, "as well as all words with a sentimental or 'sob' tinge." Lecturers were also urged not to overstress the horrors of venereal disease (which might cause an undesirable reaction), not to make the lectures too long, and not to preach. Nor were they to dwell upon such topics as women's anatomy and masturbation, or to state opinions on "social evil" (prostitution) that were at variance with government-approved policies of repression.[62]

The syllabus emphasizes that the purpose of sex is not for selfish pleasure, but for marriage and reproduction. Continence is healthy and not unmanly. In fact, outside of marriage, continence is the most normal sex life. Continence was touted as the only sure prevention against venereal disease, with all other preventatives being uncertain. Exercise, recreation and healthy mental pursuits could help a man to keep his mind off sex. Soldiers were reminded of their duty to keep fit for service, and that contracting a venereal disease was practically always a man's fault. Every "loose woman" is dirty. Soldiers had a right to demand a "clean girl" for a wife, but in turn they should be ready to give an equally clean record. Syphilis and gonorrhea and their effects were explained, and the treatment of these diseases was discussed. Soldiers were warned against seeking treatment from quacks or self-medications.[63]

Among the motion picture films used in sexual hygiene instruction, *Fit to Fight*, produced by the CTCA in cooperation with a film corporation, stands out. Unlike typical health education films of the time, *Fit to Fight* was not done in a documentary or lecture format. It was a full-length, dramatic motion picture, following the story of five draftees and their encounter with venereal disease. Each of the men has a different experience and presents a specific moral lesson. The young men are drinking bootleg liquor in a town near their training camp when they are approached by prostitutes. Four of the men enter a brothel with the prostitutes, only Billy declining. One of the

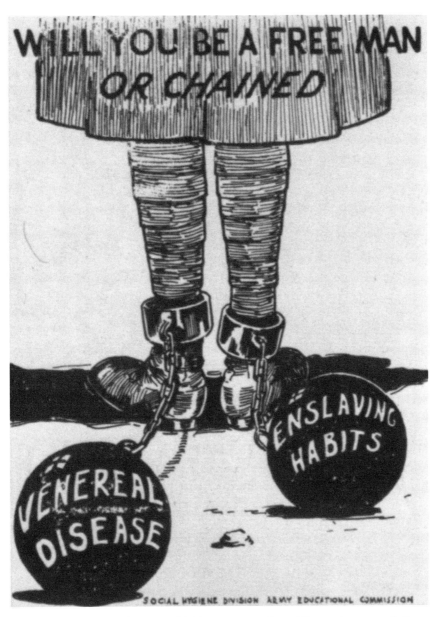

United States Army Social Hygiene Division poster warning soldiers against venereal disease and "enslaving habits" (masturbation), 1918 [Courtesy of the National Library of Medicine].

men leaves after sharing a kiss with the prostitute, but still develops a syphilitic lesion on his lip. The other three men have sexual intercourse with the prostitutes, and one develops gonorrhea and one contracts syphilis. The third of these draftees promptly obtains prophylactic treatment and is spared a venereal disease. Although Billy is at first teased for refusing to have sex with a prostitute, eventually the other men come to see the wisdom of his choice and convert to his clean-living approach.[64] As Sue Sun Yom has argued:

> While entirely masculine in his physique, socializations, and behaviors, the character of Billy lives according to a Victorian ideal of chastity and virginity verging on the stereotypically feminine . . . His character was the visible marker of a profound role reversal that had as its ultimate aim the moral prophylaxis of male soldiery.[65]

In addition to educating soldiers about the dangers of venereal disease, the CTCA recognized the need for educating civilians, both men and women. In the spring of 1918, the Social Hygiene Instruction Division (whose name was changed to the Army and Navy Section) became part of a broader new entity, the Social Hygiene Division. Headed by Dr. William F. Snow of the ASHA, the new Division was charged with expanding venereal disease education efforts from the military to the civilian population. For example, in coordination with the United States Public Health Service, the Division launched a campaign for combating venereal disease in industrial plants. Industry was important to the war effort, and venereal disease in essential war workers would interfere with the nation's military capabilities. One CTCA official emphasized that it was just as important for the "industrial army" to be fit as the army in the field. The cooperation of employers was sought in the execution of this plan. The program involved the posting of placards in plants, the placing of slips in pay envelopes, the distribution of literature, medical examination and treatment if necessary for employees who believed they had a venereal disease, and similar measures. Male employees were warned of the risks of having sex with prostitutes or "loose women."[66]

The CTCA inaugurated a related but separate educational program for female employees, "with their special needs in mind." Employers who had women on their payroll were urged to cooperate. The government claimed that women generally had no clear knowledge of venereal disease, and so instruction on this subject was necessary. A CTCA letter to employers noted that the government was fully aware of the moral issues involved, but "it is attacking the problem from the health point of view, believing that this is the most effective appeal and one which has hitherto received too little emphasis." As in the case of the program for men, the CTCA provided placards, pay envelope enclosures, and other forms of educational literature. Firms were also encouraged to consider establishing a clinic, or to make use of plant doctors and nurses.[67]

The CTCA also released a film, *The End of the Road*, in 1918 that was aimed at women. The script was written by Katharine Bement Davis, who directed the CTCA's Section on Women's Work, part of the Social Hygiene Division. The film tells the story of two seventeen-year-old women living in New York, Mary and Vera. The beginning of the film foreshadows the different paths that each will follow with the melodramatic words: "Two roads there are in life. One reaches upward toward the land of perfect love. The other reaches down into the Dark Valley of despair where the sun never shines." Mary, whose mother has educated her about sex, works as a nurse. When her old boyfriend, who is about to go off to war, asks her to have sex with him, she refuses. Vera, whose mother has not given her any sex education, works in a department store. She has sex with her lover and contracts syphilis from him. Vera consults the doctor for whom Mary works, Dr. Bell, and he shows her the effects of syphilis in hospital patients. Frightened by what she sees, Vera undergoes successful treatment for the disease. At the end of the film, the virtuous Mary marries Dr. Bell. The film is unusual for its time in that it is a man who spreads the disease to a woman rather than vice versa.[68]

Nancy Bristow has summed up the educational work of the CTCA with the civilian population as follows:

> Mirroring the efforts with the soldiers, the civilian education program employed multiple methods to reach the American population with its message of sexual purity. Pamphlets such as *VD—U. Boat No. 13!* And *Smash the Line* targeted the civilian population as a whole, whereas more directed pamphlets such as *To Girls in Wartime—A Message from the American Government* and a second feature-length film, *The End of the Road*, targeted young women and girls specifically. Traveling exhibits and lecturers, too, spread the CTCA's social hygiene message throughout the population.[69]

ISSUES OF RACE

As Bristow has pointed out, African Americans were drafted into the armed forces in World War I during a period of heightened racial tension. Although racial friction and violence was of course not new to the United States in 1917, a series of riots nationwide in the summer of that year had stoked racial animosity. While racial violence had long been associated with the South, the large-scale migration of blacks to the North in the early part of the twentieth century had made the issue of race relations a serious problem in the North as well. In this atmosphere, the War Department decided to adopt a policy of segregation among the troops.[70]

The Army training camps and related facilities were concentrated in the South, with just under two-thirds of these bases located in that region of the country. Many white southerners were opposed to the encampment of large numbers of African American soldiers in the South, fearing the possibility of armed rebellion by these troops. They argued for the organization of black troops in small units, preferably based in the North. An incident on August 23, 1917 in Houston, where a number of black soldiers stationed at a nearby camp attacked a white community and killed sixteen white civilians, flamed these fears. The Houston riot was the result of tensions arising from the refusal of black soldiers, unused to blatant discrimination in the North, to accept restrictions involving segregation on street cars and in theaters. Police arrested and sometimes beat black soldiers, eventually leading to the explosive situation on August 23. Four black soldiers also died in the riot, and sixteen of the troops involved were court-martialed and executed. Forty-three others were sentenced to life in prison. The War Department decided on a policy of distributing the black draftees throughout the camps, in both the North and South, avoiding the concentration of African Americans at any one camp.[71]

The Army's decision to adopt a policy of segregation for the troops created problems for the CTCA. Because the CTCA was committed to providing social and recreational facilities for all of the troops, they were required to set up separate programs for segregated units of blacks and whites in the same camp. Although entertainment and recreation was provided without discrimination as to race in some northern camps, this was not the case throughout the South and in some camps in the North. Speaking of the situation regarding "the presence of colored troops in southern communities," Fosdick informed the Secretary of War that efforts would be made to provide "wholesome leisure time activities for the colored troops in the same way that we do for the white." He added, however, that in so far as possible, black and white soldiers would be kept in separate sections. "In other words, the race segregation system will be carefully observed." He also appeared to view the situation concerning the reception of black troops in the South through rose-colored glasses, writing to the Secretary:

> In every case the spirit of the southern people has been fine. They do not seem to look upon the coming of the colored people with dread, but instead, feel they can handle the problem and are quite willing to undertake it, and to give both their time and money to it.[72]

In spite of Fosdick's optimistic assessment, the situation was not free of racial tensions, and the CTCA had only limited success in implementing its programs for blacks, both in the camps and in the surrounding communities. For one thing, white communities sometimes strongly protested the encampment of black troops in the camps in their area. Another problem faced by the CTCA was that the communities near some of the northern camps had only a small number of African American citizens, making it difficult for the CTCA to arrange community facilities and activities for black troops. In one case, two representatives of the CTCA urged Fosdick to use his influence to convince the War Department to rescind an order to send 12,000 black troops from Mississippi to Camp Funston in Kansas. They argued that the black soldiers would have only a limited population of their own race to interact with in the area, and that all amusement and recreational activities in the camp would have to be duplicated for these troops. They also expressed concerns about "race feelings" in the local communities, a conviction about which they proved correct when the black soldiers were sent to the camp. In one incident, a black soldier was refused admission to a local theater on the grounds that white patrons might object. Although admitting that the soldier had a legal right to enter the theater, his commanding officer criticized him for provoking a confrontation. The officer issued a controversial bulletin urging African American soldiers to refrain from going where they were not wanted, an action that prompted protest from blacks across the nation.[73]

As a result of her detailed study of the subject, Nancy Bristow has concluded that the CTCA, due to lack of funds and lack of commitment, failed to provide adequate recreational resources for African Americans in the camps. She noted that the CTCA also only rarely reached out to African Americans in the community, as it routinely did to whites, to work with them to provide appropriate recreational facilities and activities for the black troops. Bristow also criticized the separate sex education program for blacks as disorganized and haphazard. Although the CTCA assumed that African Americans were especially ignorant about sex hygiene, its belief that they would be difficult to educate slowed the development of sex education programs for blacks.[74]

As previously noted, many white believed that blacks had lax morals and an unusually high sex drive, making them more likely to contract a venereal disease. CTCA staff frequently accepted these stereotypes, as evidenced by statements in their correspondence and reports. Documents discussing the situation with regard to moral conditions in Washington, DC, illustrate this point clearly. Fosdick, for example, commented that he believed that conditions in that city were "as clean as can be expected in any large center of population in which the negro element so largely predominates." The CTCA executive secretary, referring to conditions in southwest Washington, stated that "the problem of meeting a situation such as would naturally exist where there are twenty thousand negro women and girls, with little sense of morality dwelling in a rather congested district, is most difficult of solution."[75] A report on Washington by a CTCA representative contrasted white and black prostitutes in the city. The white prostitutes, it was reported were "not offensive." They did not "loiter on the street and annoy men," but let the men make the first advance. The writer complained that black prostitution in the city seems to have gotten out of hand, and that the women had no fear of the police. The report added:

> These black women are so bold and brazen in broad daylight that they lift their arms above their heads and beckon with their fingers to passersby. Others sit in front of their shacks on chairs and solicit, while some smile and nod their heads from windows.[76]

The CTCA also bowed to southern pressures by creating segregated facilities for the detention of white and black women who were considered a venereal disease threat. Here also African Americans faced discrimination. In many areas, particularly in the South, there were no detention homes for African Americans, so they were often just placed in jails or prison farms. The federal government appropriated money for the detention homes that was rarely used by southern communities for facilities for black women. The conditions under which African American women were incarcerated were frequently unsanitary and uncomfortable.[77]

Many whites also assumed that black men had low moral standards, and these men were thus subjected to discriminatory treatment. In some camps, for example, any black soldier returning from leave had to subject himself to chemical prophylaxis because it was assumed that he had engaged in sexual activities while away from the camp. The Army reported exceptionally high rates of venereal disease among black soldiers, but the reliability of the statistics is questionable. Alan Brandt suggests that although the venereal disease rate for blacks may have been higher than that for whites, it is likely that many Army physicians were predisposed to diagnose many ailments of African American soldiers as syphilis or gonorrhea. Brandt also pointed out other factors that may have contributed to a difference in venereal disease rate, such as the relatively poor quality of health care for blacks in the United States at the time. Miles and McBride, in a study where they argue that the syphilis epidemic in blacks of the 1920s and 1930s originated in World War I, suggested a number of reasons why more blacks than whites may have contracted syphilis during the war. They point out that black soldiers sent to Europe were more frequently support laborers, such as builders and loaders, than their white counterparts, and more thus likely to remain in port areas or near large transportation centers, where health supervision was difficult because of heavy flows of transient populations. Because the military excluded black nurses and accepted black physicians only as enlisted privates, rather than as medical officers, African American soldiers did not have access to health care or medical outreach by practitioners of their own race. Many black soldiers, presumably resentful about this situation, refused to participate in venereal disease information, screening and treatment programs.[78]

THE PUBLIC HEALTH SERVICE

The First World War also made venereal disease control a specific duty of the federal health agency, the United States Public Health Service (PHS), for the first time. The PHS traces its beginnings back to a 1798 act for the relief of sick and disabled seamen. The young American republic had seen a need to provide for the care of sick or injured seamen when American merchant ships docked in the country's ports. Using a British model, the new nation created a Marine Hospital Fund, to be administered by the Treasury Department, to establish hospitals in major port cities to treat sick and injured seamen. By the time of the Civil War, this unorganized collection of locally controlled hospitals was in dire need of reform. It was reorganized in 1870 as a centrally controlled system, known as the Marine Hospital Service, with its headquarters in Washington, DC. In the following year, the first Supervising Surgeon (later called Surgeon General), John Maynard Woodworth, was appointed to run the Service. Woodworth created a mobile cadre of career physicians in uniform who could be assigned to facilities as needed, formalized by legislation in 1889 as the Commissioned Corps.

By the late nineteenth century, the Marine Hospital Service had also expanded its responsibilities to include such public health activities as quarantine and the medical inspection of arriving immigrants. As the new century dawned, the Service was becoming increasingly involved in programs for the control of disease, and was renamed the Public Health and Marine Hospital Service in 1902, and finally the Public Health Service (PHS) in 1912.[79]

The PHS was involved with venereal disease in a limited way before World War I. For one thing, marine hospitals routinely treated seamen with syphilis or gonorrhea In addition, syphilis was one of the diseases for which arriving immigrants could be excluded from the country, and so it was one of the diseases that PHS physicians looked for in the medical inspections at Ellis Island and other ports of entry. When the United States entered World War I, the Service also cooperated with the states and with the CTCA in venereal disease control work. It was the passage of the Chamberlain-Kahn Act of July 9, 1918, however, that created a separate Division of Venereal Disease (DVD) in the PHS. The newly established Division was provided with an initial appropriation of $200,000 for its operation and also given funds to be allotted to state health departments for their use in venereal disease control work. As previously mentioned, the act also provided funds, under the auspices of an Interdepartmental Social Hygiene Board, for the maintenance of the detention homes for women[80]

The duties of the new DVD, as specified in the act, were to investigate the cause, treatment, and prevention of venereal diseases, to cooperate with state boards or departments of health in the prevention and control of venereal diseases within the states, and to control and prevent the spread of these diseases in interstate traffic. Dr. Claude C. Pierce was placed in charge of the Division. With the aid of the DVD, almost every state soon made provision for the control of venereal infections as a part of the work of the state health department. By June 1919, 227 clinics for the treatment of venereal disease had been organized through the country. The PHS also launched a venereal disease education campaign in cooperation with state health departments at this time. Ralph Williams, in his history of the PHS, related how an earlier effort in 1908 by the Surgeon General of the Service to published a simple pamphlet on venereal disease had been rejected by the Treasury Department, the institutional home of the PHS at the time, on the grounds that it was not sufficiently dignified to bear the imprint of the Department.[81]

When the war ended on November 11, 1918, the DVD had existed for only a few months, so its contributions to the war effort were very limited. However, the PHS and its venereal disease program, established during the war, have played a major role in the federal government's venereal disease control program ever since. Without the impetus of the wartime emergency, however, the federal and local governments reduced funding for venereal disease programs after the armistice. It was only with the appointment of Thomas Parran as PHS Surgeon General in 1936 that a vigorous campaign to combat syphilis was once again initiated in the United States.

FOUR

"CONGRESS APPARENTLY THOUGHT THE SPIROCHETES OF SYPHILIS WERE DEMOBILIZED": THE INTERWAR YEARS

AFTERMATH OF WAR

The signing of the armistice on November 11, 1918 ended World War I. With the end of hostilities, venereal disease became less of a pressing concern for the federal government, and those who had hoped that the wartime programs would have a lasting influence on this problem were disappointed. The pronouncement of Public Health Service Surgeon General Rupert Blue in 1918 that the country had now been awakened to the dangers of venereal disease, so that the control of this "great national menace" would gradually increase until it was no longer a major problem, turned out to be overly optimistic.[1]

Over the next few years, the Commission on Training Camp Activities (CTCA) was dismantled. Its leaders, however, hoped that they could implement a demobilization strategy that would help them achieve their goal of ensuring that the influence of their work would outlive the war. Therefore as the Commission demobilized, those in charge tried to establish the Commission's work as a permanent feature of the military. Bristow has pointed out that although the CTCA was generally successful in finding successors for its work, the groups that took over its programs (such as the recreation activities) did not always share the original intentions of the Commission.[2]

The Division of Venereal Disease (DVD) of the Public Health Service, the Interdepartmental Social Hygiene Board (ISHB), and the American Social Hygiene Association (ASHA) took over and continued the social hygiene education program of the CTCA in the postwar period. However, the ISHB, created during the war by Congress to play a significant role in the fight against venereal disease, lost its funding and ceased to exist by 1922, in spite of the objection of social reformers. With the dismantling of the CTCA as well, the Public Health Service (PHS) thus became the primary federal agency involved with venereal disease in the civilian population.

The armistice heralded the end of the relatively open wartime discussion about venereal disease. Newspapers and magazines no longer publicized the problem. The New York State Board of Censors, in a ruling upheld by the courts, suddenly declared the wartime film *Fit to Fight* (renamed *Fit to Win* and shown under the auspices of the PHS after the war) obscene. The Pennsylvania Board of Censors banned any film that even used the words "venereal disease." By 1922, the PHS withdrew all of its antivenereal disease films from circulation. Brandt has pointed out that while there was a distinct increase in sexual activity during the 1920s, the so-called Roaring Twenties, "a strong crosscurrent of demand for moral rectitude and gentility persisted." In this atmosphere, he noted, "sexually transmitted diseases were drawn once again behind a veil of secrecy."[3]

One of the objections to *Fit to Win* by the Catholic Church and many social reformers, including the ASHA, was its advocacy of chemical prophylaxis (the use of chemicals to cleanse the genitals after sex in an effort to prevent venereal infection). Conservative social hygienists believed that encouraging this method of protection would lead to an increase in promiscuity. Although motivated by moral concerns, they pointed out that anything that promoted promiscuity would inevitably lead to an increase in venereal disease. Many state and local health boards, whether or not they believed in the efficacy of prophylaxis, did not promote it because of public opposition to the practice. Even PHS Surgeon General Hugh Cumming was not in favor of education about and provision of prophylaxis, arguing in 1927 that those persons who were most irresponsible and therefore most in need of protection would not have the foresight to use it.[4]

The use of condoms was rarely mentioned by public health officials or social hygienists during the 1920s and 1930s. Sexual abstinence was the main means of prevention of venereal disease promoted in education campaigns. The relationship of condoms to birth control complicated the picture. The ASHA, for example, fearful of alienating its Catholic constituents, avoided the issue of birth control entirely. In one 1940 letter to a colleague, ASHA Executive Director Walter Clarke discussed the advisability of not being drawn into a fight over birth control. He voiced his belief "that if we proceed cautiously we may continue to avoid battles on this touchy subject."[5]

Even Thomas Parran, who headed the PHS's DVD in the 1920s and became one of the nation's most prominent antisyphilis campaigners when he succeeded Cumming as PHS Surgeon General in 1936, was largely silent on the issue of condoms, in spite of his desire to emphasize public health over morality considerations in the fight against venereal disease. As suggested by Brandt, it may be that Parran, a Catholic, had pushed his morality to the breaking point in his venereal disease campaign and could not go any further on the question of prophylaxis. We shall have more to say about Parran's views on prophylaxis later in the chapter. As Brandt also noted, unwanted pregnancy and venereal disease had long been viewed as means of controlling sexuality, and many social reformers worried that condoms and birth control would "take the fear of these potential consequences out of sex" and "risk a breakdown of restraints on family and society."[6]

This conservative approach is reflected in the sex education campaigns for boys and girls initiated by the PHS following the war, which have been described in detail by historian Alexandra Lord. The program for boys between the ages of 12 and 20, entitled "Keeping Fit," was launched in 1919, in part out of a concern for the level of venereal disease in the country. The PHS partnered with the Young Men's Christian Association (YMCA) in this effort.

Separate programs were eventually developed for white boys and for African-American boys, although the latter program was not developed until relatively late in the campaign. The heart of the program was an exhibit of forty-eight panels, as well as a lantern slide version, although pamphlets were also published and lectures arranged. Although designed primarily with sex education in mind, the exhibit covered a broad array of health subjects, including diet, sleep, bathing, and physical activity. Only the last segment of the exhibit discussed sexuality and disease, with an emphasis on the germs that cause venereal disease. For an exhibit that was supposed to provide education about sex, sexuality was curiously downplayed—because the PHS and the YMCA wanted the exhibit to receive wide support in the community. The exhibit did not discuss prophylaxis. As Lord described it:

> Venereal disease itself is referred to in vague and often dire terms, with women and men who engage in sex out of wedlock all being cast as carriers of the disease. There are no real explanations as to how reproduction works or what sexual maturity entails. Overall, the PHS discussion of sexuality was so elliptic that boys who lacked a prior knowledge of the "facts of life" would be unlikely to learn the basics of human reproduction from viewing the exhibit. Although remarkable by modern standards for its failure to address sexuality, the reticence displayed by the organizers of Keeping Fit was typical of most sex education campaigns during this period.[7]

The program for women did not begin until 1922, and it was even less successful than the one for boys. For one thing, the PHS partnered in this case with the General Federation of Women's Clubs, which had fewer resources than the YMCA and also found itself declining in vigor during this period. Perhaps most importantly, funding for the PHS venereal disease program was also on the wane. The campaign, moreover, promoted the persistent view that women were responsible for most venereal

infections, emphasizing that it was up to women to control the strong sexual desires
of men. According to one of the campaign's pamphlets, a woman who thoughtlessly
stimulated the emotions of a man by her words, acts or dress is "making herself
responsible for his temptation and mistakes." Women were thus divided into two
types, the clean and decent girl and the girl who aroused men's sexual instincts.[8]

The PHS was also not especially successful in another attempt to deal with sex
education as past of a series of films produced in conjunction with Bray Studios in
the 1920s. The series, which consisted of twelve motion pictures, had the general
title of *The Science of Life.* Two sex education films were included in this group—
Personal Hygiene for Young Women and *Personal Hygiene for Young Men.* Consisting
largely of titles interspersed with some pictorial material, the sex education films, not
surprisingly, focused on abstinence and control of sexual urges. They paid very little
attention to venereal diseases, with no significant discussion of the nature of these
diseases and no mention of any form of prophylaxis. According to the producer, while
"The Science of Life" series was widely shown in American schools, the films on sex
hygiene were not well received by school authorities, who believed that the parent
(rather than the teacher) should instruct children about sex.[9]

As noted above, funding for the PHS DVD also declined dramatically during the
1920s, decreasing from $4 million in 1920 to less than $60,000 in 1926, the year in
which Thomas Parran became head of the Division. When he took over the DVD,
it seemed like a dying operation. The situation only worsened with the onset of the
Depression in 1929.[10] As the Division's federal budget decreased, so did the money
made available to the states for venereal disease control. By 1926, all federal support
to the states for venereal disease work was withdrawn. Years later, Parran looked back
on this period and wrote:

> Congress apparently thought the spirochetes of syphilis were demobilized with the
> army. More accurately, no further thought whatever was given to syphilis, and this first
> national public health effort came to an untimely end.[11]

But the spirochetes had not laid down their arms and the problem of syphilis and
other venereal diseases continued into the 1920s. The most frequently cited figures
by the early 1930s suggested that about one in every ten Americans suffered from the
disease. The reliability of syphilis statistics was still in question, however, and critics
also charged that these figures were exaggerated by antisyphilis crusaders in an effort
to instill fear in the public. In fact, by the late 1930s, when better statistics were
becoming available, estimates began to be revised downward. Even the ASHA, which
was one of the groups accused of attempting to frighten the public through inflated
statistics, had reduced its estimate of syphilis incidence to 5 percent. One PHS study
in 1938 reported a syphilis rate of 1 percent for the country as a whole.[12]

Many social reformers tended to blame the apparent rise in venereal disease after World War I on the liberalized sexual morality of the 1920s rather than on decreased public health efforts. Newer and more sexually explicit dances, jazz, the automobile, and other aspects of the decade worried moral reformers. Brandt has noted that "[s]ocial hygienists who had ultimately been more concerned with preserving sexual ethics than preventing disease could not countenance the changes they observed."[13]

The main private agency concerned with venereal disease, the ASHA, believed that with the end of the war it had "before it a greater opportunity and a larger responsibility than in any previous stage of its existence." However, financial problems threatened its effectiveness. A significant amount of its budget during the war had been provided by the Surgeon General of the Army, but it was obvious to the leaders of the ASHA that this source of funding would soon disappear. The Association turned to John D. Rockefeller and his Bureau of Social Hygiene for support, and was rewarded by a commitment from the Bureau to contribute to the ASHA $2 for every dollar raised by the Association, up to a maximum of $100,000. This support allowed the Association to continue its educational and investigative activities.[14]

A report of the ASHA's activities for 1922–1923 provides some idea of the programs of the Association during this time period. The ASHA listed among its achievements for this fiscal year a study of social hygiene literature in libraries designed to supplant unreliable publications with those that were more scientific, a conference of religious leaders to encourage the integration of social hygiene in their work, lectures at numerous colleges and other educational institutions, the publication of several books and pamphlets (as well as the Association's *Journal of Social Hygiene*), a survey of social hygiene legislation in the United States, investigations of vice conditions in twenty-four cities, the preparation of two new exhibits, loans of motion pictures, and cooperation with various agencies and institutions (including the PHS) interested in social hygiene.[15]

With the advent of the Depression, the ASHA feared that the disruption in traditional family roles and economic hardships would lead to increases in prostitution and venereal disease. The Depression took its toll on the Association as well, resulting in significantly reduced contributions and consequent budget cuts. Nevertheless, the ASHA managed to continue many of its programs, in part through cooperative efforts with more than fifty different organizations. The Association continued to send undercover agents to investigate commercialized prostitution in response to requests from local officials, although a tight budget limited the number of these surveys. The analysis of these surveys showed that the number of "red light" districts in cities, which had declined during the 1920s, experienced an alarming increase by 1933. Comparing that year to 1928, the ASHA found that those cities which it had given a "good" rating dropped from 19 to 11, while those which had earned a "bad" rating increased from 11 to 28.[16]

During the early 1930s, the ASHA cooperated with the Canadian Social Hygiene Association to advise on the film *Damaged Lives*, produced by Weldon Pictures Corporation, and served as the sponsor of the motion picture in the United States. The film tells the story of Donald, a young man from a good family who, "influenced by too many high-balls and a series of incidents for which he is in no way responsible," yields to temptation and has sex with an alluring woman. Donald is later told by this woman that she has discovered that she has a venereal disease, and she eventually kills herself in despair. Donald goes ahead and marries his sweetheart Joan, although he does go to a quack doctor whose advertisement he sees in a "cheap newspaper" because of his concern that he may have contracted the disease. The quack reassures him that he is fine. When Joan becomes pregnant, however, blood tests by their family doctor reveal that she and Donald are infected with syphilis. Donald at first denies his illness, but then accepts the facts and undergoes treatment. Joan is despondent and believes that all happiness is over for her, but eventually Donald restores her faith in the future. "The story ends on a high note of confidence."[17]

Damaged Lives was released in 1933, and apparently included as an epilogue a twenty-minute lecture following the one-hour narrative story. Reviews tended to give the production a low rating as far as entertainment was concerned, but admitted that it was a frank and absorbing discussion of a social problem. Reviewers also apparently found nothing obscene or morally objectionable in the film. One reviewer noted that the audience was very attentive and that they applauded at the end of the lecture epilogue. When it was shown in Baltimore in 1934, over 65,000 people, one-tenth of the city's adult population, saw the film. However, the film was originally banned in New York State, and not shown until 1937, when the New York Regents overruled the New York State Censors. Thomas Parran, serving as New York State Commissioner of Health at the time that the film was originally released, later criticized the decision to ban it in the state, calling *Damaged Lives* "an excellent moving picture" that "was in no way offensive to good taste or to the principles of pedagogy."[18] This incident reflects the continuing hesitancy to discuss venereal disease openly in the United States during this period.

THERAPY FOR SYPHILIS

As previously discussed, Paul Ehrlich's discovery of the arsenical drug Salvarsan in 1910 represented a major breakthrough in syphilis therapy. Along with the isolation of the spirochete that caused the disease and the development of a diagnostic test for it, Salvarsan led to increased optimism about the prospects for controlling syphilis. At the Rockefeller Institute for Medical Research in New York, syphilis became a major area of study. Scientists recognized that a better understanding of the disease would certainly enhance the chances of developing a successful vaccine or better therapeutic agents against syphilis. One of the Rockefeller researchers, Hideo Noguchi, published the results of experiments on lutein, an inactive solution of the syphilis spirochete, which produced a specific skin reaction. Noguchi believed, in the words of Susan Lederer, "that his success in growing pure cultures of the treponeme [spirochete] and the discovery of a specific skin reaction were critical steps in the search for a serum that would cure syphilis." He expected the lutein skin test to serve as a complement to the Wasserman blood test in the diagnosis of syphilis. After a number of animal tests to determine the safety and utility of the lutein test, he initiated a clinical study involving four hundred patients.

The lutein test did not meet Noguchi's expectations. However, his use of normal (i.e., nonsyphilitic) patients, including children, as controls in his experiments was controversial. He was criticized, especially by antivivisectionists, for introducing into the bodies of children the loathsome germs of syphilis, even if, as he argued, these were dead germs. The hospital superintendents and physicians involved in providing Noguchi with access to the patients were also denounced by these critics. Efforts to bring charges against Noguchi for subjecting healthy children to the lutein test without their consent or the consent of their legal guardians were unsuccessful because the Manhattan District Attorney's Office declined to prosecute Noguchi.[19]

A few years later, the Rockefeller Institute once again became embroiled in a controversy involving syphilis and human experimentation. In 1916, a University of Michigan researcher, Udo Wile, published a paper in the *Journal of Experimental Medicine*, which was affiliated with the Rockefeller Institute and edited by its director, Simon Flexner. Wile's research involved performing brain punctures on patients with neurosyphilis. His goal was to determine whether or not active spirochetes could be found in the brain of individuals with neurosyphilis, in which case introducing antisyphilitic drugs directly into the brain tissues might prove to be an effective treatment.

Although Wile argued that the brain puncture was a simple and painless procedure, critics charged that the operation entailed risks and possible pain as well. In addition, the neurosyphilitic patients involved were suffering from paresis (a condition involving brain damage and characterized by dementia and paralysis) and were in no position to grant permission as they were essentially insane. No attempt had been made to obtain the consent of a guardian or relative either. Once again, antivivisectionists played a prominent part in the attack on Wile. Some physicians and scientists criticized Wile's experiments, but they did so cautiously and gently for fear that their comments might be used by antivivisectionists in their crusade against animal and human vivisection research. The ethics of human experimentation also became an issue, as we shall soon see, in the Tuskegee Syphilis Experiment that began in the early 1930s.[20]

Salvarsan (arsphenamine), or the related and more soluble, easier to administer compound Neosalvarsan (neoarsphenamine), often combined with mercury, remained the preferred treatment for syphilis during the period of World War I. Initially the length of treatment generally extended from several weeks to perhaps two months. Treatment regimens varied, however, and the high cost of the drug meant that there was a tendency to stop its use once the Wasserman test, measuring the presence in the blood of the spirochete that caused syphilis, was negative. As a result of experience during the war and immediately thereafter, however, it became clear that it was necessary to continue treatment for a significantly longer period of time in order to avoid relapse.

In 1921, the use of bismuth to enhance the efficacy of the arsenicals was introduced. Like arsenic and mercury, however, bismuth had certain toxic side effects. During the 1920s, the standard therapy for syphilis involved weekly injections of arsenic preparations, frequently rotated with mercury and bismuth compounds, for a period of one to two years. In the United States, the most widely accepted schedule was that developed by the Cooperative Clinical Group, organized in 1928 by five large American syphilis clinics. Their protocol for acute syphilis involved weekly injections of Neosalvarsan and bismuth, on an alternating schedule, for a period of sixty-eight weeks. This regimen was complicated to administer, expensive, prolonged, and potentially dangerous, and patients did not always complete the full course of therapy.[21]

Although this therapy was reasonably effective in the treatment of primary and secondary syphilis, side effects ranged from relatively minor ones, such as nausea and headache, to serious problems such as necrosis (death of skin cells) at the site of injection, kidney failure, and acute hepatitis, occasionally resulting in death. In addition, arsenical therapy had little or no effect in cases of advanced neurosyphilis, a late stage of the disease affecting the nervous system. The ineffectiveness of the drug was especially pronounced in patients whose neurosyphilis had progressed to the point where they had developed general paresis.[22]

In 1917, however, an Austrian physician began experimenting with a form of therapy for paresis that became widespread in the 1920s and after. A medical graduate of the University of Vienna, Julius Wagner-Jauregg accepted an appointment in a psychiatric clinic in 1883. Although he had no formal training in psychiatry, which was still in its infancy as a discipline, he became professor of psychiatry at the University of Graz in 1893. He also continued clinical research in mental health in his hospital practice. Early in his career, he developed an interest in investigating the effects of inducing fevers in patients with psychoses, based on empirical observations from early times that patients with mental illness sometimes seemed to improve when attacked by a fever.

In 1917, Wagner-Jauregg decided to try using malaria as a form of fever therapy in patients with paresis. He injected nine patients suffering from this condition with tertian malaria, a form of the disease that was relatively innocuous and could generally be cured by drug therapy with quinine. He found that six of the cases showed significant remission, and in three of these cases the remission proved to be enduring.

In 1919, he began this experimental treatment on a large scale. Others also began to carry out clinical trials with malaria therapy, which appeared to be far more successful than any previous treatment for paresis. In 1922, the treatment was used on the first American patient at St. Elizabeth's Hospital in Washington, DC. The method was soon widely accepted and Warner-Jauregg received the Nobel Prize in Physiology or Medicine in 1927 for his discovery of the therapeutic value of malaria inoculation in the treatment of paresis.[23]

Joel Braslow has argued that we cannot answer the question of whether malaria fever therapy actually worked with any degree of certainty. No randomized clinical trails of the sort that would be accepted as evidence today were ever performed on the method. With the discovery of the effectiveness of penicillin against syphilis in 1943, malaria therapy was eventually phased out, although it remained the treatment of choice until the late 1940s and early 1950s, and continued to find some use even after that time. In its heyday, it was certainly widely believed to be effective. In addition, Braslow has pointed out that it resulted in a decided improvement in the relationship between physicians and paresis patients. Whereas previously, both the patients and their doctors had viewed the condition of the patients as hopeless, there was now some cause for optimism. Braslow wrote:

> The advent of malaria therapy restructured patients' and physicians' perceptions of themselves and each other. Irrespective of whether the treatment worked, not only did these physicians believe that they could act decisively against the syphilitic spirochete, but their belief in its efficacy allowed them to write more sympathetically about their patients and, perhaps, to care for them in a less objectified and more humane way. Furthermore, this new technology not only allowed patients to seek hospitalization voluntarily but permitted even those who were there against their will to become active participants in their treatment.[24]

Developments in the 1930s resulted in some modifications in the treatment of syphilis in its earlier stages. As Kampmeier has pointed out, the stumbling block to adequate treatment with arsenicals continued to be the issue of compliance on the part of the patients. A course of weekly injections for over a year was too much of a burden for many patients, and so often the full treatment was not carried out. Experiments reported by Harold Hyman at Mount Sinai Hospital in New York in 1933 demonstrated that active medications could be delivered relatively safely by means of slow intravenous drip. This work led Hyman's colleague Louis Chargin to speculate that the intravenous drip procedure might be applied to arsenic therapy, with the possible result of curing syphilis in a matter of days or weeks, instead of a year or more. However, the procedure required hospitalization of the patients.

Chargin, Hyman, and their coworkers began clinical testing of the intravenous drip method of Neoarsphenamine therapy for syphilis at Mount Sinai Hospital in 1933.

Although the results were promising, the death of a patient led the team to look for a drug that might be less toxic and more stable. At about this time, other investigators had shown that Mapharsen (arsenoxide) was much less toxic than Neoarsphenamine but equally as effective. The Mount Sinai group switched to Mapharsen and continued their studies with good results and a substantial decrease in toxic effects in a five-day treatment regimen. Large-scale clinical trials at a number of institutions confirmed these early results, demonstrating that at the most effective dose intravenous Mapharsen therapy yielded satisfactory results in 85 to 90 percent of cases of primary syphilis and 70 percent of cases of secondary syphilis. The availability of this technique led to the development of the Rapid Treatment Centers in World War II that will be discussed in the next chapter.[25]

Of course, there was also no shortage of quack doctors and patent medicines supposedly able to cure syphilis, as had been the case for centuries. In nineteenth century America such nostrums as Swaim's Panacea and Helmbold's Extract of Buchu had been advertised as cures for syphilis.[26] So-called medical or anatomy museums, generally aimed at men, also were often fronts for quacks who claimed to treat venereal disease and sexual dysfunctions. Brooks McNamara described a typical museum of this type as follows:

> Once inside the main room, the assault on the patron's nerves began in earnest. Everywhere about him were glass cases filled with hideously diseased organs modeled in death-like wax or luridly painted papier-mâché. The lights were low, the atmosphere hushed and funereal. Case after case displayed gaping sores and hideous deformities attributed to syphilis, gonorrhea, or that nameless terror of the nineteenth century, the "secret vice," masturbation . . . At this point a solicitous "floor man" would appear from nowhere and begin to talk to the frightened patient. If it appeared that the customer was in need of medical aid—or could be convinced that he was—he was steered upstairs to the "medical institute" run by an "eminent specialist" in the various secret diseases.[27]

In the twentieth century, as regulation of the advertising and labeling of medicines increased at both the state and federal level, the marketers of syphilis remedies turned to using euphemisms for the disease in an attempt to disguise their claims. Everyone knew, for example, that "blood poisoning" in an advertisement meant syphilis. Products sold as "blood purifiers" had been used by some people as remedies for syphilis in the nineteenth century. Sarsaparilla tonics, such as Ayers and Hoods, were popular in this regard, as this plant (as we have seen) was originally thought to be a remedy for syphilis. Such products continued to be used in the 1920s and beyond. For example, Compound Syrup of Sarsaparilla and Burdock with Iodide of Potassium was being sold as a treatment for "blood poisoning resulting from syphilis" in the 1930s.[28]

By the late nineteenth century, however, sarsaparilla had largely fallen into disuse for this purpose in orthodox medicine, although syrup of sarsaparilla was still being used as a vehicle for delivering drugs such as mercury and iodine (that were used to treat syphilis). Textbooks of pharmacology of the early twentieth century generally dismissed the value of sarsaparilla as a remedy for syphilis. Arthur Cushny's popular textbook of pharmacology, for example, stated that the drug "has some reputation in the treatment of syphilis, but there is no reason to believe that it is of any service here."[29]

Patent medicine quacks were not hesitant to don the mantle of science to sell their wares. Not long after Ehrlich discovered Salvarsan, for example, a New York charlatan marketed a cure for "blood poison" (syphilis) in which he used both Ehrlich's name and the number 606 (a term by which Salvarsan was also known). In the 1930s, a practitioner opened the "606 Medical Laboratory" in Chicago for the treatment of "men's disease"—a euphemism for syphilis and gonorrhea. The advertisement for this establishment could easily have given one the impression that Dr. Ehrlich himself was in charge. Another twentieth century "cure" for syphilis was named Ricord's Specific, drawing on the name of a famous nineteenth-century syphilologist.[30]

Dr. Sayman's Wonder Herbs was another patent medicine of the twentieth century that supposedly cured syphilitic "taints." The remedy consisted of a mixture of various plant products, such as ginger, rhubarb, licorice, and senna, along with sodium bicarbonate or sodium carbonate. The Chief of Drug Control of the Food and Drug Administration noted in 1933 that while the medicine might be of some value in relieving gas in the stomach and bowel, it was worthless in the treatment of syphilis. Furthermore, he added:

> Yet this concoction was recommended for syphilitic "taints," as if you could have just a little bit of this dread disease! But when you have syphilis you have it. It is as impossible to have a mere taint of it as it would be to fire off a cannon a little bit at a time."[31]

Quack devices were also used for the supposed diagnosis and cure of syphilis. Albert Abrams, "the dean of twentieth century charlatans," built a series of machines that he claimed could diagnose the disease of a patient from a sample of dried blood, even if the patient were miles away. In time, Abrams stated that the patient's autograph would work just as well, which supposedly enabled him to diagnose syphilis in famous persons of the past such as Henry Wordsworth Longfellow and Edgar Allan Poe. A New York "clinic" used an electrical device to treat young men who had been led to believe that they might be infected with syphilis. The patient sat naked on a kind of toilet throne with his back against a metal plate and his scrotum suspended in a whirling pool of liquid. Both the liquid and the metal plate were hooked to a battery, and the patient received a shock, presumably convincing him that the treatment was working.[32]

The shame associated with syphilis and the prolonged and unpleasant treatment offered by orthodox medicine continued to prompt many Americans with the disease to turn to patent medicines and quack doctors in the postwar period. The fact that in many cases of syphilis the early symptoms are sometimes light and generally temporary as the disease goes into a latent phase led many people to believe that they had indeed been cured by these remedies or "doctors." In 1937, Thomas Parran summarized this problem:

> Moreover, quacks flourish and the sale of patent medicines for syphilis has become big business because even the severe and recognizable early symptoms usually are transitory. No matter what nostrum is taken; no matter how inadequate the treatment given, eventually these early signs and symptoms of the disease disappear. When they disappear, thousands of syphilis victims think themselves cured, not realizing that instead of cure, this marks the end of the period when the best chance for it is possible.[33]

Syphilis patients may also have turned to self-medication when they could not afford to see a doctor. A full course of therapy by a private physician could cost anywhere from $300 to as high as $1,000 in unusual cases. In an effort to resolve this problem, the PHS worked with the states to help them establish public clinics to treat venereal disease. By 1923 more than 500 such clinics had been established, and they had treated nearly 600,000 patients. The clinics were not always free, but even when they charged, the cost was a fraction of that of treatment by a private physician.[34] The PHS itself maintained a clinic for the treatment of venereal disease in Hot Springs, Arkansas. The clinic was created in cooperation with the National Park Service of the Department of the Interior, which operated Hot Springs National Park. In 1926, one PHS office wrote that the clinic "offers free treatment to paupers and during the past year 3,075 patients there received 32, 315 treatments." The clinic also carried out research on venereal disease and served as a training center for medical officers from the states.[35]

But with the Depression, funding for venereal disease decreased, and the number of persons seeking free or inexpensive treatment for syphilis increased substantially. It has been estimated that demand at public health clinics rose by at least 20 percent between 1929 and 1933. Brandt stated that:

> According to estimates of the New York State Division of Social Hygiene, fully one-half of all newly infected cases now sought treatment at public expense. Health economists Leon Bromberg and Michael M. Davis argued that eighty per cent of the population could not afford the cost of adequate care for syphilis from private physicians.[36]

THE TUSKEGEE SYPHILIS STUDY

African Americans, especially in inner cities and in the rural South, were one of the groups that did not have sufficient access to health care for syphilis. Many whites viewed blacks as a particularly "syphilis-soaked race," with an excessive sex drive and low morals, which further complicated access to treatment. In the early twentieth century, some public health officials were becoming more convinced of the importance of environmental and social factors in promoting disease. They began to devote more attention to the health needs of the underprivileged. In this context, some became concerned about the problem of syphilis in the African American community and the lack of available treatment. This concern was based on a variety of motives, from a genuine belief in the importance of providing health care to all, to a paternalistic "white man's burden" attitude, to a fear that syphilis in the black community posed a threat of spreading to the white community.[37]

In the late 1920s, the PHS's DVD carried out a survey of the rate of syphilis among black plantation workers in Mississippi. Their results on more than 2,000 workers tested indicated a syphilis rate of about 25 percent, a cause for concern. At about that same time, the Julius Rosenwald Fund, a philanthropic organization that supported programs to improve the welfare of black Americans, decided to expand its activities into the area of health care. The Fund appointed Michael Davis, a medical reformer, as director of medical services. Since the Fund had not previously had a medical division, Davis decided to enlist the aid of the PHS as he fashioned plans for new health programs for African Americans. He asked the PHS to appoint an advisor who would review proposals for aid that were coming in from state health officials and to recommend policies governing the Fund's health programs. Dr. Tailaferro Clark, a southerner and a PHS medical officer, was assigned to the task.

PHS Surgeon General Cumming approached the Fund with a proposal for a health project in the rural South in 1929. Cumming informed Davis about the high rates of syphilis that PHS had discovered among black plantation workers in Mississippi. He asked the Fund to support a project to provide treatment to the infected workers, to serve as a demonstration of how effective a treatment program could be. He reported that the plantation owners had agreed to cover half the cost of the treatment and Cumming asked the Fund to cover the rest. Davis agreed, although placing some conditions on the funding, including the addition of a black nurse to the project staff, since training and employment of black health care workers was one of the goals of the Fund.[38]

The Mississippi project was placed under the direction of PHS medical officer Oliver Wenger, who had been in charge of the syphilis survey of plantation workers. The treatment program, utilizing neoarsphenamine and mercury, began in the late summer of 1929. As this project neared completion, Wenger discussed with Thomas Parran, then head of the DVD, the possibility of expanding the demonstration to other areas. Parran and Clark drafted a proposal for such an expansion and sent it to the Rosenwald Fund in October 1929. The proposal was approved by the Fund the following month and scheduled to begin in 1930 in six southern counties (including the original Mississippi site).[39]

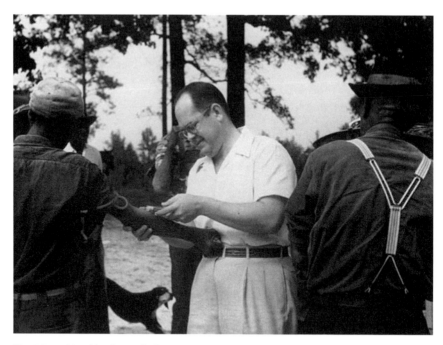

Physician taking blood sample from a patient in the Tuskegee Syphilis Study, which began in 1931 [Courtesy of the National Archives and Records Administration].

One of the sites selected was Macon County, Alabama, an area that was severely economically depressed. The PHS survey revealed an incredible rate of syphilis of 36 percent in that county. In the spring of 1932, its stock suffering from the effects of the Depression, the Rosenwald Fund decided that it could not continue the syphilis control program, involving treatment of those infected. In fact, the program had already been abandoned in Macon County in August of the previous year because the state of Alabama, also suffering financial woes as a result of the Depression, was not able to meet the Rosenwald Fund's cost sharing requirements. These were the circumstances leading up to the Tuskegee Syphilis Study—good intentions that resulted in a bad project.[40]

The best book on the subject is still James Jones' *Bad Blood: The Tuskegee Syphilis Experiment*, first published in 1981 and reissued in an expanded version in 1993. More recently, Susan Reverby has edited a volume of essays and documents entitled *Tuskegee's Truths: Rethinking the Tuskegee Syphilis Study*. Numerous articles have also been written on the history, ethics, and impact of the study, some of which are reprinted in Reverby's volume.[41]

By the time that the Rosenwald project ended in 1932, Taliaferro Clark had succeeded Parran as head of the DVD. In compiling a final report on the syphilis demonstration, Clark apparently conceived of the idea of a new experiment that would cost the PHS relatively little money, unlike a large-scale treatment program. It occurred to him that the conditions were perfect in Macon County for a study of how syphilis progressed in African Americans when it is left untreated. The syphilis rate had been shown to be exceptionally high in the county, and most of those infected had never received any treatment. Therefore there would be a large population on which to draw for a study of untreated syphilis.

James Jones is convinced that Clark would have preferred to carry out a treatment program in Macon County, but since it did not appear that there would be funds for such a program in the foreseeable future, he decided that perhaps he could salvage something from the abandoned project. Much was already known about the natural history of syphilis, but Clark believed there was still much to learn, especially with respect to the progress of the disease in blacks. A large-scale study of untreated syphilis had been carried out earlier on whites in Norway, and the PHS believed it would be useful to have a similar study done on blacks. At the time, it was widely believed in the medical community that syphilis in blacks was very different from the disease in whites. For example, many physicians believed that syphilis was more likely to attack the nervous system in whites and the cardiovascular system in blacks. Once the study had begun, at least one PHS physician involved expressed an interest in seeing similar research carried out with other racial groups, such as American Indians. In addition, the Norwegian study had raised questions about whether everyone suffering from latent syphilis benefited from the available treatment, thus suggesting another aspect of the disease that could be investigated.[42]

Jones claims that Clark did not initially expect the study to last for more than six months to a year, and did not plan on denying treatment to anyone for longer than that. Clark also assumed that the subjects of the study would not have the means to afford treatment, and public or charitable funds for this purpose were not available, so they would be left untreated in any case. He recognized, however, that there were other risks to the subjects, for example the discomforts and dangers to which they would be subjected as a result of the spinal tap to obtain the spinal fluid needed to diagnose neural syphilis.[43]

PHS leaders sought and were relieved to receive the cooperation of the Tuskegee Institute and its John A. Andrews Memorial Hospital, located in Macon County, in the study, thus bringing African American educators and health workers into the project. Administrators at Tuskegee apparently thought that federal attention to the poor health conditions of blacks in the county would help the institution get more funding for its programs. Eunice Rivers, an African American nurse working at Tuskegee and at Andrews Hospital, was employed by the PHS for the study and came to play a vital role as the liaison between the PHS and the men who served as subjects of the experiment.[44]

The PHS also secured the approval of the state health officer, but only on the condition that some treatment be provided to the men. The level of treatment, however, was minimal. Syphilitic patients were supposed to receive eight doses of neoarsphenamine (Neosalvarsan) and some additional treatment with mercury. PHS medical officer Raymond Vonderlehr was sent to Macon County to select the subjects, who were to be black males between the ages of 25 and 60, and to oversee the field work. In addition to the commitment to the state health officer, Vonderlehr also provided some treatment to most of the patients at first because he believed that it would help keep them in the study through the point of the painful spinal tap. In fact, the promise of free treatment was used to attract subjects into the study. PHS officials decided that the low level of treatment involved would not significantly affect the course of the disease in the men and hence not invalidate the results of the study, whereas Jones has argued that it was a fatal flaw that made the study useless from the point of view of studying the effects of untreated syphilis. Jones also described the haphazard way in which treatment was administered:

> All the men in the study received treatment. The quantity and the form depended upon when the patient was examined, what drugs happened to be on hand at the moment, and whether the patient was too old or too ill to be given both neoarsphenamine and mercury. Moreover a drug shortage hampered the study throughout the winter and spring.[45]

Although the experiment was scheduled to end, Vonderlehr decided to continue it when he succeeded Clark as head of the DVD in 1933. Vonderlehr believed that following these cases for at least another five or ten years would yield valuable knowledge about the course and complications of untreated syphilis. Various inducements, such as free meals and transportation on the days of examination, were offered to the men to maintain contact and keep them in the study. The men had already been deceived in certain ways about the study, for example, by being told that the spinal tap was a "special free treatment," and this deception continued and even increased when the study was extended. The men were made to believe that they were continuing to be treated for their condition, but they were actually given medicines that had no effect on syphilis, such as aspirin. In fact, during the length of the study, the PHS made efforts to ensure that the men would not receive treatment for syphilis from other sources. For example, the names of the study subjects were circulated to Macon County physicians with a request that these men be referred back to the PHS if they sought care. The men were also not told that if they accepted the free hospital care that they were offered if they became severely ill, their bodies would be subject to autopsy if they died in the hospital. To further persuade them to come to the hospital if they were seriously ill, the PHS offered to cover their burial expenses, using a grant from the Milbank Memorial Fund.[46]

Even when increased funding became available to the PHS for syphilis control through the Social Security Act of 1936 and the National Venereal Disease Control

Act of 1938, the Service continued the Tuskegee Study. In 1937, the PHS initiated a mobile trailer syphilis clinic in three counties in southeastern Georgia, aimed at providing blood tests and treatment for rural African Americans. The men in the Macon County experiment, however, continued to receive no treatment. Throughout Thomas Parran's national campaign against syphilis, discussed below, the study continued. Even after the introduction of penicillin as a much safer and more effective treatment for syphilis in 1943, the subjects of the Tuskegee Study remained untreated. Discussions of the ethics of human experimentation prompted by the revelations about Nazi medical experiments at the Nuremberg Trials at the end of World War II also had no impact on the Tuskegee syphilis experiment. In fact, the study continued for forty years.

Although the PHS had reviewed the study several times over the decades, the decision had always been made to continue it. As Jones has noted, there were few detractors and many supporters of the study in the PHS. If anyone did challenge the experiment, defenders pointed out how much the PHS had invested in the study and how valuable the scientific results would be.[47] One PHS officer, clearly recognizing the controversial nature of the study, even suggested in 1950 that the PHS could utilize the fact that many of the patients had received some therapy for the disease "for the specific purpose of allaying some of the apprehension that normally is manifested by individuals who hear about the United States Public Health Service conducting a study of untreated syphilis, particularly in this day and age."[48]

The experiment was not kept secret, however; thirteen articles describing the research were published in medical journals over the years. It is doubtful, however, that the general public had any awareness of the study. Then in July 1972 Jean Heller of the Associated Press broke the story in the press, utilizing information provided by Peter Buxton, who had worked for the PHS in the 1960s as a venereal disease interviewer and investigator in San Francisco. Buxton was concerned about the study and had raised questions about it with PHS officials since 1966. In 1972, discouraged by getting nowhere in his efforts to get the PHS (for which he no longer worked) to discontinue the study, he talked to a longtime friend who was with the Associated Press in San Francisco. She turned over the documents that Buxton provided her with to her superiors at the Associated Press, and eventually the story was given to Heller, an investigative reporter who worked for the Press' research bureau in Washington, DC.[49]

The criticism that followed the public disclosure of the study led the Department of Health, Education, and Welfare (DHEW), the administrative home of the PHS, to form the Tuskegee Syphilis Study Ad Hoc Advisory Panel on August 28, 1972. The nine-member panel, which included five African Americans, was asked to decide whether the study was justified in 1932, whether the subjects had given their informed consent, and whether penicillin should have been given to the men when it became available. The panel was also asked to determine whether or not the study should continue and to assess current policies concerning human experimentation. Their final report was issued in April 1973. The report concluded that the experiment was "ethically unjustified" even when it was begun in 1932 and that it was scientifically unsound with results that were meager compared to the risks to the human subjects involved. The panel also made policy and procedural recommendations for improving the protection of human subjects in experimentation. Allan Brandt has argued that the report failed to identify all of the ethical problems with the study. For example, he has pointed out that while the report does state that the PHS did not obtain "informed consent" from the patients, it fails to make clear (with the exception of a minority opinion submitted by Jay Katz) that the PHS actually lied to the men. Brandt also concluded that the panel did not sufficiently focus on the racism inherent in the study.[50]

By the time that the Ad Hoc Advisory Panel issued its report, the federal government had finally ended the Tuskegee Syphilis Study and authorized treatment of the subjects. In July 1973 a lawsuit was filed on behalf of the study participants and a settlement was reached in December 1974 whereby the government agreed to pay about ten million dollars in compensation to the participants or their heirs. On May 16, 1996, President William J. Clinton offered a formal apology to the survivors of the study and their families in a ceremony at the White House. The distrust of public health authorities today by many African Americans is a continuing legacy of the study.[51]

Racist attitudes about blacks clearly contributed to the Tuskegee Syphilis Study. Jones has noted that it is ironic that the PHS officials who approved and carried out the study had a serious interest in the health of African Americans. The PHS had been involved in a number of programs involving the health of blacks since the 1920s, including serving as the "working arm" of National Negro Health Week. Although it may seem difficult to believe now, Jones also claimed that by the standards of the 1930s the PHS physicians associated with the study were "racial liberals" and "truly progressive." Vonderlehr and Wenger, for example, "promoted black hiring and used their influence repeatedly to arrange attractive residencies for young black physicians and to secure advanced medical training in the nation's leading medical schools for older black staff members."[52] Jones did not contend, however, that these men were free of racial bias. They shared many of the stereotypical views of the day about the superiority of whites over blacks. In discussing the racial views of many public health officials of the day in general, Jones wrote:

> Health officials did not discard racial prejudice; they simply did not let their racism blind them to their professional duties. Compared with the real black-baiters of the day, however, the racism of these health officers was mild. Their prejudices took the form of paternalism.[53]

Yet Jones clearly criticized the unethical practices of the Tuskegee Syphilis Study and surely recognized that in this case racism did blind the health officials involved to their professional duty. As physicians and public health workers, their first duty should have been to place the welfare of their patients above their research interests. Patients should not have been exposed to unnecessary risks and deceived into believing that they were receiving treatment rather than serving as human subjects in an experiment.

The racist attitudes of PHS officials of the day are clearly illustrated in remarks that they made. Wenger, for example, was amused by what he called the childlike reactions of black patients, made reference to "cotton-patch negroes" who rarely took a bath and slept in their filthy underwear, and used the term "darkeys" to describe blacks. Clark referred to the African Americans in the study as being very ignorant and easily influenced by things that would seem to be of minor importance to a more intelligent group, and he questioned the logic of "over-educating" blacks to create "what we might call white-collared Negroes, with nothing to do but get into mischief."[54]

In an article published in 1939, Leroy Burney, who was in charge of the PHS mobile syphilis clinic for rural blacks in that period and who was later to serve as Surgeon General, exposed his biases concerning African Americans. For example, he noted that "as promiscuous as these people are," it is difficult to track down the source of infection. He also suggested that the "moral code" of the African American might not be as stringent as that of whites. He also claimed that blacks were slow to learn about venereal disease, and complained that available educational films about the problem were "not simple and plain enough for them to understand." Other PHS staff members at the time expressed similar concerns about the difficulty of producing a good film on venereal disease that was "at the proper intellectual level" for black audiences, stressing the need for "utter simplicity" in such a production.[55]

Even Thomas Parran, while arguing in 1937 (when he was serving as Surgeon General) that the white man introduced syphilis into the black community and that the high syphilis rate in that community was largely due to lack of education and poor living conditions, accepted some of the myths surrounding the racial aspects of the disease. He believed that syphilis was indeed a very different disease in blacks than in whites, with the blood vessels in the African American being particularly susceptible to the disease, "so that late syphilis brings with it crippling circulatory diseases, cuts his working usefulness in half, and makes him an unemployable burden on the community in the last years of his shortened life." Parran also believed "that the colored woman remains infectious two and one-half times as long as the white woman." He also allowed that it might be true, although not the whole truth, that sexual promiscuity accounts for the increased prevalence of syphilis among blacks. He did note, however, that promiscuity tends to be more common in any community of the underprivileged, whether black or white. As Surgeon General, Parran also continued the PHS support of the Tuskegee Syphilis Study.[56]

THOMAS PARRAN AND THE NEW CRUSADE AGAINST SYPHILIS

In 1936 the campaign against syphilis was rejuvenated with the appointment of Thomas Parran to succeed Hugh Cumming as Surgeon General of the PHS. As previously mentioned, Parran had served as the head of the PHS's DVD in the late 1920s. Parran was born on September 28, 1892 and raised on his family's tobacco farm near St. Leonard's, Maryland. He obtained his undergraduate education at St. John's College in Annapolis and earned his M.D. degree from Georgetown University in 1915. During his medical school years, he spent two summers working as a volunteer in the health laboratory of the District of Columbia under Joseph Kinyoun, who had earlier in his career served in the PHS. From 1887 to 1899, Kinyoun served as the first director of the Service's Hygienic Laboratory, which was later to evolve into the National Institutes of Health. Under Kinyoun's influence, Parran joined a PHS field team building sanitary privies and surveying rural health conditions in the South in 1917. That same year he became a member of the PHS Commissioned Corps.[57]

Parran spent the next nine years on a number of assignments for the PHS, most of them involving rural health, sanitation, and communicable disease control. In 1926 he obtained his first leadership position when he was appointed chief of the PHS Division of Venereal Diseases. Parran shifted the Division's emphasis from areas such as sex education toward more scientific pursuits such as research, health surveys, and treatment demonstrations.[58]

As previously noted, the budget of the DVD had been slashed by the time Parran became its head, and he may not have been sorry to leave it in 1930 to become state health commissioner for New York. He remained a PHS commissioned officer, but was loaned to the state at the request of Governor Franklin Delano Roosevelt. In announcing the appointment, Governor Roosevelt said that in addition to his own immediate knowledge of Parran's qualifications and training, he had received endorsements of his choice from eminent physicians and health organizations. Roosevelt noted that:

> I regard the administration of the office of commissioner of health of such paramount importance, affecting the health and lives of the people of this state, that I have not the slightest hesitance in going outside the confines of the state to find the man with the special training and capacity for this position.[59]

Not surprisingly, Parran made the control of syphilis one of his priorities for New York. He managed to obtain increased appropriations for this purpose, with the goals of providing more diagnostic and treatment facilities, improving case reporting and investigation of contacts, and increasing professional and public education about the disease.[60] In 1934, Parran came to national attention because of an incident involving a radio broadcast. Parran was scheduled to speak about "Public Health Needs" on the Columbia Broadcasting System (CBS) on November 19, 1934. In reviewing his script, CBS objected to a section where he mentioned syphilis and asked him to delete it. Parran replied that he would give either all of the speech or none of it, and so the broadcast was cancelled and replaced by a musical program. Parran also resigned from the public health committee of the National Advisory Council on Radio in Education in protest.[61]

The cancellation received coverage in the newspapers and was denounced by social hygiene and public health leaders. William Snow of the ASHA, for example, wrote to both the president of CBS and the president of the National Advisory Council on Radio in Education complaining about the fact that Parran was not permitted to mention syphilis on the air. Upon learning of Parran's experience, John Rice, Health Commissioner of New York City, also wrote to CBS, as well as to the National Broadcasting System (NBC) and fifteen newspapers, protesting the censorship. About a month earlier, Rice had himself suffered a similar fate. An address that he was giving at a Kiwanis Club luncheon was being broadcast on NBC, but he was abruptly cut off the air when he began discussing syphilis.[62]

In responding to Rice's letter, the president of NBC argued that radio broadcasters have to be careful about what they allow on the air because they receive a good deal of criticism from parents who believe that their children should not hear information on certain topics no matter how important they may seem. He explained that people tend to view radio as an invited guest in their homes, and that remarks that might be made in a lecture hall or book or magazine article without offense might not be appropriate for radio. NBC had even turned down many laxative advertisements, he claimed, because "the mere statement of the performance of laxatives has brought forth so much condemnation from radio listeners." In another case, the general manager of a radio station in Milwaukee, when asked for his opinion of whether or not the word "syphilis" should be used on the air, suggested "that it would be more proper to use the phrase 'a social disease' instead of the word 'syphilis' due to the fact that a radio stations has as its' audience many children of tender years and the use of the latter word might cause considerable embarrassment to certain parents because of their inability to explain it to children if questioned." He added that adults would understand perfectly what was meant by "social disease" but that his experience with children had shown that this term causes no questions in their young minds.[63]

By the time that Hugh Cumming retired in 1936, Roosevelt had become president of the United States, and he turned to Parran to succeed Cumming as PHS Surgeon General. Roosevelt had already appointed Parran in 1934 to serve on the Committee on Economic Security, the group that drafted the Social Security Act of 1935. Parran

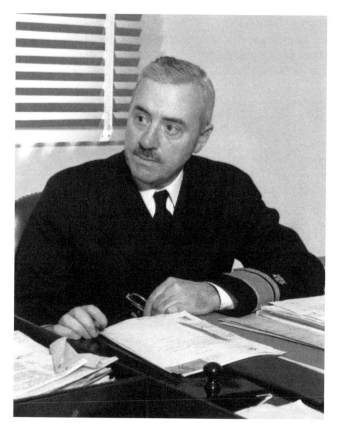

Thomas Parran during his tenure as Surgeon General of the United
States Public Health Service (1936–48) [Courtesy of the Centers for
Disease Control and Prevention].

was sworn in as Surgeon General on April 6, 1936. He lost little time in launching a
new national campaign against syphilis, which was in full swing by the fall of 1936.[64]

One of Parran's first salvos in his war against syphilis was an article that he
wrote entitled "The Next Great Plague to Go." It was published in July 1936 in both
Survey Graphic and *Reader's Digest*, the latter of which had about 500,000 subscribers.
Breaking the conspiracy of silence, Parran argued that it was time to talk about syphilis
in the open. One of the major obstacles in the fight against syphilis in the United
States, he claimed, was the view that nice people do not have syphilis, nice people
do not talk about syphilis, and nice people do not have anything to do with syphilis.
The article contained pictorial graphs that dramatically illustrated the magnitude of
the problem.[65]

Parran's visits to Scandinavia in 1926 and 1935 had impressed him with how these
countries handled the venereal disease problem. He especially admired the way in

which the venereal diseases were treated like other diseases and openly discussed. In Denmark, for example, he noted that with respect to syphilis, "Nobody minds talking about it; nobody is either horrified or fascinated by it." The Danes, he reported, were amused by the inhibitions of Americans when it came to discussing venereal disease. Compared with his own radio experience in 1934, the Scandinavian attitude must have seemed refreshing to Parran. It was not only the openness with which syphilis and other venereal diseases were discussed, however, that made the Scandinavian countries models for the control of these diseases. Stringent reporting requirements, the availability of free clinics, and the respect for medical authority in these countries all contributed to their relatively low rate of venereal disease.[66]

In 1937, Parran published his landmark and popular book, *Shadow on the Land: Syphilis.* The book was aimed at a general audience and was intended, the author said, to express the disease's "impact upon the nation and its relationship to contemporary public health and other public problems."[67] The subjects covered included a description of the disease and its modes of transmission, its history, methods of control in the United States and selected other countries, prostitution, and other topics, including a proposed platform for action. Parran's action recommendations fell under three headings: locate syphilis (diagnosis), obtain public funds that assure adequate treatment for all infected persons, and educate the private physician and general public. The book included the kinds of illustrative material that had appeared in Parran's earlier articles, and it ended on the following encouraging note:

> If we could and would go a step farther—as far as the Scandinavians have gone—syphilis need no longer threaten your children and mine. All of us working together can make it a rare disease in our day and generation. And when it is done, we will all wonder why so simple a thing was not done long before.[68]

In this last remark, Parran was not implying that eliminating syphilis would be an easy task. Rather he was stressing that we have the scientific and medical means at hand to do the job. Physicians and public health workers know how to diagnose the disease, how to prevent its spread, and how to treat it. It was not the limits of medical science that was preventing the eradication of the disease. There were no serious differences among authorities, he pointed out, as to how to combat the disease. Parran believed that if Americans overcame their "ostrichlike attitude" toward syphilis and devoted sufficient resources to the problem, then the disease could indeed be eliminated.

Overly moralistic attitudes, he contended, could interfere with the efforts to fight venereal disease. Parran emphasized that he was heartily in favor of movements designed to prevent syphilis by moral prophylaxis, the teaching of sex hygiene, and the elimination of prostitution. But while this kind of long-term campaign was being carried out, it was crucial to act now and use the medical means available to stop the syphilis plague.[69] In a 1937 article in *Reader's Digest*, he emphasized again the importance of educating the public "to remove all stigma of shame and turpitude from the syphilitic sufferer," adding that:

> Not until we have stripped the disease of its traditional moral implications can we make headway against it. We must think of syphilis scientifically as a dangerous disease, which it is, rather than moralistically as a punishment for sin, which it often is not.[70]

In spite of his call for openness in speaking about venereal disease, Parran said relatively little on the subject of prophylaxis, as previously noted. In her book on the Chicago Syphilis Control Project, Suzanne Poirier, although giving Parran significant credit for his antisyphilis efforts, criticizes him for placing too much emphasis on moral prophylaxis and too little on other methods of prevention of venereal disease. Although there is some justification for her arguments, I think that she has overstated the case. In *Shadow on the Land*, Parran does specifically discuss condoms and chemical prophylaxis, though it is true that he raises questions about their effectiveness. And while he supported moral prophylaxis, he also clearly believed that health agencies had to deal with venereal diseases as dangerous contagions and leave the teaching of sexual morality to the home, the church, and the school. In a letter written in 1944, he explained that it should be possible, using available scientific methods, to eradicate these diseases in our lifetime, a timetable that "may be well in advance of any major changes in the sex habits of the population as a whole." Given his desire to work with social hygiene organizations such as the ASHA, as well as his Catholic background, it is not surprising that he did not make mechanical and chemical prophylaxis a mainstay of his campaign. He did, however, attempt to remove the moral stigma from venereal disease and he focused on the use of available scientific methods, such as testing, case finding, health education, and treatment, rather than moral exhortations, to stem the tide of venereal disease. When the stakes were raised as the United States entered another world conflict, the PHS under Parran also did devote more attention to prophylaxis, as we shall see.[71]

Parran's efforts succeeded in breaking down the social taboo against discussing syphilis openly in the popular press. Newspapers and magazines began broadly publicizing the problem of venereal disease. Parran was featured on the cover of *Time* for October 26, 1936 when the American Public Health Association met in New Orleans and the Surgeon General was installed as the Association's new president. The magazine noted that breaking down the taboo on the discussion of syphilis and tackling the disease "scientifically rather than morally is the high and burning purpose in the official life of the Surgeon General."[72]

Parran was of a more activist bent than his predecessor as Surgeon General and he expanded the programs and services of the PHS and raised the priority of public health on the national agenda as a part of Roosevelt's New Deal. To him, venereal disease was the most pressing public health problem, and he devoted significant effort and resources to fight it. In December 1936 he organized a National Conference on Venereal Disease Control to set the agenda for this battle. President Roosevelt became the first president to address the question of venereal disease directly when he sent a message to the Conference indicating his support and assuring attendees that the "Federal Government is deeply interested in . . . reducing the disastrous results of venereal disease."[73]

One of the resolutions adopted by the National Conference was to call upon Congress for a substantial increase in funds to fight venereal disease, especially to support efforts in the states. Under the Social Security Act, some $10 million had already been earmarked to the PHS for this purpose, about half of which was to be used to aid the states. The Conference asked Congress to provide an additional $15 million. Early in 1938, Senator Robert LaFollette of Wisconsin and Congressman Alfred Bulwinkle of North Carolina introduced legislation to provide increased federal aid for the eradication of venereal disease. The LaFollette-Bulwinkle bill was passed and signed into law by President Roosevelt on May 25, 1938 and known as the National Venereal Disease Control Act. It authorized a total of $15 million over the next three fiscal years, to be administered by the PHS, for venereal disease control. A statement issued by the PHS said that "it would make possible for the first time a simultaneous and planned attack against syphilis in forty-eight States." As Brandt has pointed out, this act was typical of other New Deal welfare legislation in looking toward a national solution, expanding the role of the federal government into areas previously seen as being within the domain of the states.[74]

The legislation provided for federal grants through the PHS to state boards of health to develop methods for controlling venereal disease. Funds could be used to set up diagnostic and treatment facilities and to provide necessary training for personnel. The act also supported research on the treatment and prevention of venereal disease. According to Brandt, the National Venereal Disease Control Act of 1938 had a substantial impact on the venereal disease problem in America.

By 1940 the effects of programs that the federal funding helped to establish could be partially measured. Clinic facilities for the treatment of venereal disease had grown from 1,750 in July 1938 to almost 3,000 in July 1940. Moreover, the improvement and expansion of existing treatment centers had also served to make therapy more accessible. The $15 million appropriation helped to provide private practitioners with diagnostic and epidemiological services, as well as with free drugs when necessary to assist in the treatment of disadvantaged persons, and in some cases for all their patients regardless of income. As a result of the increase in facilities and public subsidies, the number of patients receiving the minimum required therapy jumped from 15 to 58 percent.

Another indication of the value of the legislation was the fact that the number of blood tests performed to detect syphilis increased by some 300 percent between 1936 and 1940; funds from the Act helped to make the necessary diagnostic facilities available.[75]

The encouragement of blood tests as a diagnostic measure for identifying the presence of syphilis was an important arm of the antivenereal strategy. During this period, requirements for premarital and prenatal blood tests became common. Although most states had laws prohibiting marriage where one party had syphilis, these laws were laxly enforced and easy to circumvent. Most required merely a note from a physician or an affidavit signed by the groom, since the laws generally applied only to men, attesting to the fact that he was free from syphilis. In 1935, however, Connecticut became the first state to require a blood test and physical examination of all prospective brides and grooms before granting a marriage license. If one of the parties was infected, the license would not be issued until that individual could be shown to be noninfectious. Other states soon followed. By 1940, a total of twenty states required premarital blood tests for syphilis for both the prospective bride and groom. In 1938, three states passed the first laws requiring blood tests of expectant mothers, and by 1940 a total of nineteen states had such legislation, thus contributing to a decrease in the incidence of congenital syphilis.[76]

Parran's campaign also emphasized case-finding, the tracking down of an infected individual's sexual contacts, and then testing and, if necessary, treating them. Unfortunately, many people suffering from a venereal disease were hesitant to identify their sexual partners. Private physicians, concerned about the confidentiality of the doctor-patient relationship, were also reluctant to report cases of venereal disease that they treated to public health officials. As Brandt has stated, "Venereal disease posed the fundamental dilemma of individual privacy versus the public good, a conflict that remains largely unresolved."[77]

Perhaps the earliest full-scale local campaign launched as a part of Parran's nationwide effort was that of the city of Chicago, inaugurated on January 18, 1937, less than a month after the national conference held in December 1936. Suzanne Poirier has written a detailed account of the Chicago Syphilis Control Program, a program that the PHS itself viewed as a specially concentrated effort that could hopefully serve as a model for the rest of the nation. Local, state, and federal officials cooperated in the program, and the Chicago *Tribune* provided the necessary publicity. One of the mainstays of the campaign was the push to get the public to volunteer for free blood tests for syphilis. Free drugs would also be provided for those who required treatment. Leaders referred to the effort to reach as many people as possible, including those who might not know they had the disease, as a "syphilis dragnet," using a term borrowed from other PHS public health campaigns. The Chicago board of health mailed a survey to a million households, asking people if they were willing to have themselves and their families tested for syphilis. A march on August 13, 1937, where marchers carried banners with slogans such as "Friday the 13th is an Unlucky Day for Syphilis," was one of the most dramatic events designed to draw attention to the testing program.[78]

Even the Federal Theatre Project, part of the New Deal Program for the arts and funded by the Works Progress Administration, became involved in the campaign. On April 29, 1938, the Chicago unit of the Theatre Project opened a run of thirty-two performances of a play by Arnold Sundgaard entitled *Spirochete*. The play traced the history of syphilis, as well as dealing with contemporary issues surrounding the disease, such as the then relatively new Illinois law requiring premarital blood testing for syphilis. Surgeon General Parran and prominent science writer Paul De Kruif had reviewed the script for accuracy. As part of its historical account, the play recounts the then widely accepted view that Columbus and his men brought the disease back from the New World to Europe. In later productions of the play the Columbus character was identified only as a nameless sea captain because of protests by the Knights of Columbus against the association of their namesake with syphilis. During intermission, patrons could obtain free blood tests for syphilis in the theater lobby.[79]

The production of *Spirochete* also fit in with another major strategy of the venereal disease campaign, namely, education of the public about syphilis and gonorrhea. The PHS issued films, pamphlets, posters, and other materials designed to inform the public about the dangers of venereal disease, its modes of transmission, how to prevent it, and the importance of seeking diagnosis and treatment if one suspected that he or she might be infected. This educational campaign increased significantly after the United States entered World War II, as discussed in the next chapter.

FIVE

"FOOL THE AXIS—USE PROPHYLAXIS": SYPHILIS IN WORLD WAR II

AMERICA PREPARES FOR ANOTHER WORLD WAR

On September 3, 1939, World War II began with the declaration of war against Germany by France and Britain in response to Hitler's invasion of Poland two days earlier. Although the United States quickly expressed its neutrality, the country became increasingly concerned over the coming months about the worsening situation in Europe and about Japanese actions in the Pacific. Just five days after the declaration of war in Europe, President Roosevelt proclaimed a limited national emergency. By the spring of 1940, the United States was offering some support to Britain and was beefing up its military preparedness. On September 16, 1940, the country instituted its first peacetime program of compulsory military service.[1]

As the nation prepared for the possibility of involvement in another world conflict, concerns about the impact of venereal disease on the war effort increased. Recognizing the need to cooperate with civilian authorities in a venereal disease campaign, as they had during World War I, military leaders met early in 1940 with representatives of the PHS and the ASHA to plan a joint strategy. These conferences led to the preparation of a resolution that was commonly known as the "Eight-Point Agreement," a plan that was also adopted by the Conference of State and Territorial Health Officers in May 1940.[2] The points agreed upon were the following:

1. early diagnosis and adequate treatment by the military of enlisted personnel infected with venereal diseases;

2. early diagnosis and treatment of civilian populations by local health departments;
3. reporting by military medical officers, where possible, of probable sources of infection of servicemen to state or local health authorities;
4. reporting by local or state authorities to military medical officers of contacts of enlisted men with infected civilians;
5. recalcitrant infected persons with communicable syphilis or gonorrhea should be forcibly isolated during the period of communicability;
6. decrease as much as possible opportunities for contact with infected persons;
7. aggressive program of education in military and civilian populations;
8. public and military officials desire the assistance of ASHA and other voluntary welfare organizations in developing and stimulating public support for the above measures.[3]

As in past wars, military and public health leaders believed that prostitution would be a major source of venereal disease. In spite of pressure from the military, the PHS, and groups such as the ASHA, however, it was becoming obvious by late 1940 that law enforcement officials in many communities were not successfully repressing prostitution. On January 20, 1941, therefore, Congressman Andrew May introduced a bill to prohibit prostitution near military establishments and to empower the Secretaries of War and of the Navy, as well as the Federal Security Agency (the home department of the PHS) "to take such steps as they deem necessary" to suppress prostitution and prevent the violation of the act, accepting the cooperation of local authorities. Violations of the law would be punishable by a fine of not more than $1,000 and/or imprisonment for not more than one year. The law clearly stated that the military and the Federal Security Agency were not given "any authority to make criminal investigations, seizures or arrests of civilians charged with violations of this Act," but making such crimes a federal offense allowed a federal law enforcement agency such as the Federal Bureau of Investigation to intervene if necessary. The officially titled May Act was passed and became effective July 11, 1941. Although the May Act was invoked only twice during the war, in Tennessee and North Carolina, it served to push local authorities to rid their communities of prostitution so that the federal government would not step in.[4]

In spite of this spirit of cooperation, the May Act ultimately led to a tense situation between the PHS and the military. In the fall of 1941, Thomas Parran and Raymond Vonderlehr published a book entitled *Plain Word about Venereal Disease*. In the book, they chastised the military for not taking sufficient action to protect soldiers against venereal disease, especially with respect to prostitution around Army camps and other facilities. The authors complained that the military was not making use of the May Act, and called upon the Army and Navy to enforce the provisions of the law. Parran and Vonderlehr did not mince words, stating that it was "treasonable to waste manpower."[5]

Understandably the military was not happy with this stinging criticism from the Surgeon General of the PHS. Neither was the President, who was especially annoyed at comments on the book's jacket, which criticized the federal government's apathetic policy toward the problem. Federal Security Administrator Paul McNutt, Parran's boss, reprimanded the Surgeon General and warned him not to repeat what he called an "unethical and untactful procedure." There were some who came to the Surgeon General's defense, such as Raymond Fosdick, former head of the CTCA, and the *American Journal of Public Health*, and Parran stood his ground. The entire controversy soon evaporated, however, when the Japanese bombed Pearl Harbor on December 7, 1941. The time for internal bickering was over as the United States entered the war.[6] In retrospect, one of the authors of the official history of the Army Medical Department during World War II credited the publication of *Plain Words about Venereal Disease* with having "expedited and enlarged efforts to suppress commercialized prostitution around military areas."[7]

VENEREAL DISEASE CONTROL IN THE MILITARY

The first question confronting the Army with respect to venereal disease was whether or not to induct men who were infected. At the beginning of the war, Army policy stated that registrants with any form of venereal disease were not acceptable for general service, although those with acute or chronic syphilis could be admitted to limited service. Since gonorrhea could be readily treated by then with sulfa drugs, the induction of registrants with this disease into general service was temporarily deferred until they had undergone treatment and been cured. After the United States entered the war and manpower needs became critical, these regulations were reviewed. In addition, public opinion was opposed to a policy that in a sense might be viewed as penalizing moral behavior by drafting those who did not have syphilis and rewarding those who did by exempting them from general service. In the summer of 1942, the Army began experimenting with inducting men suffering from venereal disease and curing them before assigning them to active duty. An estimated 200,000 men with venereal disease were eventually inducted into the Army during World War II after standards were liberalized.[8]

The wartime admission policy of the Women's Army Corps, established in 1942 on an auxiliary basis and converted to full status in 1943, was to reject women with venereal disease. Some cases slipped through the screening, especially at first because women were originally given the same physical examinations as men, without any pelvic or gynecological examination, although such an examination was soon required.

Army regulations required all personnel to continue to undergo monthly physical examinations, which included checking for signs of venereal disease. One Army surgeon pointed out that venereal disease could not easily be detected in women by a cursory inspection, and he suggested that a more complicated pelvic examination be performed every six months instead. The Surgeon General of the Army, however, decided to leave it up to surgeons at posts and field stations as to how to handle the situation. At some posts, pelvic examinations were made monthly, stirring protests from the women, who argued that the examination was uncomfortable and immodest, and often could not detect venereal disease in any case. It should be noted that almost all of the examining physicians were men. Over time, procedural changes were made to respond to some of the concerns of the women. Monthly inspection was to be simple and private. Women were to be suitably draped, and no inspections were to be made in the nude. A female company officer was to be present at all times, and inspection of the pubic hair would not be made routinely. More detailed pelvic examinations were to be made only if indicated by certain symptoms.[9]

Although no institution such as the CTCA was established by the military in World War II, many of the functions of that body with respect to vice control were carried out by other entities. The military, for example, tried to provide soldiers and sailors with "wholesome" activities to divert them from undesirable pastimes. Movies, athletics, organized entertainment, and other forms of recreation were made available to the troops in the camps.[10]

Undoubtedly the most important of the agencies in the United States that provided recreational outlets for servicemen outside of camp in their off-duty hours was the United Service Organizations for National Defense (USO), formed by six nonprofit groups in 1941. The founders included organizations that had assisted the military in World War I, such as the YMCA. The USO operated clubs and canteens for servicemen throughout the country, by 1944 assisting about one million people a day in over 3,000 sites. Although both men and women volunteered for the organization, it was women who provided the labor for most of the USO activities, especially the operation of the clubs. The USO drew largely upon white middle-class women, whom they believed were "inherently sexually respectable and feminine," thus providing female companionship of a "wholesome" sort for the men. Marilyn Hegarety, in her book on the mobilization and control of female sexuality in World War II, has discussed the efforts of government and social groups to both mobilize wartime women's patriotic sexuality (e.g., as USO hostesses) while at the same time suppressing deviant female sexuality (e.g., prostitution and promiscuity). She pointed out that the image of the sexually dangerous female and the sexually alluring female morale builder became conflated with each other, as illustrated by the coining of the gendered term "patriotute" (from "patriot" and "prostitute") by PHS physician Otis Anderson.[11]

As in World War I, the organizations operating the USO were concerned about controlling a population of young men, away from their homes and communities, who could be corrupted by unsavory influences. The USO believed that these men would miss their homes and appreciate the "taste of home" provided in the clubs and canteens, an influence that would help protect them from immorality. General George C. Marshall, Chief of Staff of the Army, argued that the military would look after the spiritual and moral, as well as physical, well-being of servicemen while they were on military grounds, but could not take responsibility for their off-base behavior. It was up to groups such as the USO to offer the men an alternative to sex and liquor in the community.[12]

The military, as they had in World War I, also initiated a campaign of venereal disease education for the troops, including pamphlets, lectures, and films. The Army education program was viewed as a continuing effort from when the soldier was inducted until he was discharged. Two Army Medical Corps officers described the program in an article as follows:

> This educational process is inaugurated at the induction station with the distribution of a brief pamphlet. At the reception center . . . he is given talks on sex hygiene and venereal disease by a medical officer, a line officer, and a chaplain. In addition, he is shown a film on the subject and given another pamphlet. At the replacement training center where the soldier's basic military training is completed, two hours are devoted to venereal disease education, employing film strips, supplemented by talks by officers. After the solider has completed his basic training and is assigned to a unit, his education in venereal disease is pursued by means of further talks at regular intervals, and by the use of additional films, pamphlets, posters and other health educational material.[13]

These officers indicated that the Army employed the factors of fear, intelligence, pride, and patriotism to motivate the men to use the knowledge they had been given to avoid venereal disease. Fear, they admitted, was the dominant theme, not only fear of the diseases themselves, but also fear of the consequences for such matters as the future health, home life, fertility, and sexual capacity of the soldier. On the other hand, they found that appeals on strictly moral grounds, urging the avoidance of illicit sexual intercourse, were "of limited value." Venereal disease education, they argued, was not "evangelism," and there was little evidence that the Army had been at all successful "in converting to continence those individuals who were promiscuous before their entry into the service."[14]

Posters and pamphlets reminded servicemen to stay away from prostitutes and "pick-ups," to use prophylaxis, to be true to their wives and girlfriends, to avoid quacks and patent medicines if they suspect they are infected, and not to let down their military buddies by being taken out of action by a venereal disease. Films, often graphic in their depiction of venereal disease, were also used to deliver the message. As one retired American serviceman phrased it, "Every soldier at some time in his basic training was forced to sit through what we used to call a 'Susie Rotten-crotch' film where a soldier is shown out meeting a local female, only to appear at sick call with gonorrhea or syphilis shortly afterwards."[15]

Perhaps the most famous and most viewed of the training films made for military personnel during the war, according to Eberwein, was *Sex Hygiene* (1941), directed

DON'T VISIT HOUSES OF ILL-FAME

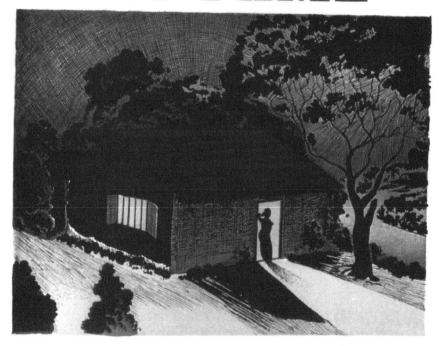

If in doubt call at the nearest Hospital
for free and confidential advice

SAVE YOURSELF & YOUR FAMILY FROM V. D.

World War II American poster aimed at soldiers and warning them against houses of prostitution. [Courtesy of the Centers for Disease Control and Prevention].

by John Ford and produced by Darryl F. Zanuck. The film tells the story of Pete, a soldier who has sex with a prostitute and contracts a venereal disease. The heart of *Sex Hygiene*, however, is a movie within a movie. Soldiers at an Army base are shown a new film about venereal disease, which includes candid shots demonstrating the use of a condom (being put on a metal rod rather than a penis) and depicting cleansing of the genitals and prophylactic irrigation of the penis after intercourse. The motion picture also makes use of graphic depictions of some of the effects of secondary and tertiary syphilis, such as ravaged skin and crippled limbs. A popular film used by the Navy, *The Story of D.E. 733* (1945), makes some of the same points, using the narrative device of the story of a group of sailors who have sex with prostitutes while on shore leave. Although they were provided with condoms by the ship's pharmacist, they neglect to use them and are infected by venereal disease.[16]

The venereal disease education and prophylactic campaign was apparently aimed largely at enlisted men rather than officers. Stan Lee, who went on to fame as the creator of Spider-Man and other superheroes, recalled that during his World War II Army service he was asked to design a poster encouraging soldiers to seek prophylactic treatment after having sex. Lee noted that his superiors kept emphasizing that the poster was aimed at enlisted men, and he added that "perhaps it was felt that, in the case of officers, no germ would dare."[17]

As shown by the above discussion of the education campaign, the military had come to the conclusion during World War II that preaching continence alone would not reduce the rate of venereal disease. As one Army medical officer stated, as quoted by Brandt, "The sex act cannot be made unpopular."[18] The Army established prophylactic stations within each command, and, where possible, in adjacent civilian communities. Condoms were also sold at post exchanges. Church groups and other civilian representatives complained to the Army about the provision of mechanical and chemical prophylaxis to soldiers, arguing that it encouraged promiscuity and undermined the case for continence, but the military stood firm on this point. In one reply to a Catholic Bishop, the Army Surgeon General commented that the War Department had no desire to minimize the importance of the moral aspects of venereal disease, but that in the interest of military efficiency the problem had to be treated like any other disease. He explained:

> It must be recognized that regardless of what advice is given an unknown proportion of men will expose themselves to the hazard of venereal contagion. For such individuals the Army advocates the use of mechanical and chemical prophylactics, not as contraceptives, but solely as an effective procedure for the prevention of infection.[19]

In the case of the Women's Army Corps, however, there was no discussion of mechanical or chemical prophylaxis in the "social hygiene" course given to the women.

Abstinence was the only means of protection discussed. Nor were condoms or chemical prophylactics provided for the women. Leaders were confident that because of the "high type of women" admitted into the Corps, such measures would not be necessary. Nevertheless, newspapers reported that there was a secret War Department policy that authorized the issuance of prophylactics to members of the Women's Army Corps, and even suggested that the women were expected by the Army to put them to good use for "morale purposes." The rumor may have gotten started because initially women who were going overseas were inadvertently given the same equipment as men, including a prophylactic kit, but this practice was quickly terminated. The newspaper reporter who initiated the story was an outspoken critic of President Roosevelt and may have let his feelings interfere with his journalistic judgment as he apparently did not confirm the facts. Secretary of War Stimson issued a statement proclaiming that the charges were absolutely false.[20]

Issues of race as well as gender confronted the military. The Army inducted large numbers of African Americans during the war, but made the decision to continue to uphold segregation. The War Department argued that it was not its job to try to alter American customs, and that it had to focus on fighting a war. Therefore separate units continued to be organized for blacks and whites. Ironically, in spite of the insistence on segregation, white officers were often placed in charge of black units.[21]

The Navy, meanwhile, had eliminated almost all African Americans from its service in the period between the wars. When World War II began, there were only a few dozen blacks on active duty in the Navy other than in the messman branch (involved with preparation of meals). A committee was created by the Navy in 1941 to consider the question of inducting blacks. A majority of the committee believed that enlisting blacks (other than as mess attendants) would lead to "disruptive and undermining conditions." The committee also reported to the Secretary of the Navy that the enlisted personnel of the Navy were representative of all citizens of the United States "within the limitations of the characteristics of members of certain races." In other words, the committee believed that very few African Americans would be fit to serve in the Navy and Marine Corps. The Navy continued to resist expansion of the number of blacks for some time, justifying this policy by arguing that this type of discrimination was part of a larger pattern in the country, where the white race believed it was superior, did not wish to admit blacks to intimate family relationships, and would not accept blacks in positions of authority. As the war progressed, however, the Navy was forced to admit larger numbers of African Americans, although limiting the roles that they could play and maintaining segregation.[22]

Racist attitudes were also reflected in venereal disease policies in the military. We have already seen that many stereotypes existed in American society about black sexuality and promiscuity. Such perceptions were reinforced for many by the evidence that the rate of venereal disease for black inductees and soldiers was eight to twelve times that of whites. One PHS survey reported that of the first two million draft board examinations among men 21–35 years of age, the rate of syphilis among the black selectees was 25.2 percent as opposed to 1.7 percent for white selectees. Although the official history of preventive medicine in the Army during World War II admitted that the causes for this high incidence of venereal disease in black troops were "basically socioeconomic," the reasons given in the history for the differential rates in selectees could allow much of the blame to be placed on the black community. The factors cited are low educational level and general lack of knowledge about health care, inadequate law enforcement in black communities, and lack of recognition among blacks about the seriousness of the problem together with reluctance to face the facts. The history did acknowledge, however, that insufficient recreational facilities for blacks in civilian areas near camps, an Army venereal disease education program "inadequate to meet the specific needs" of black soldiers, and a "defeatist attitude" on the part of many commanding officers with respect to the prevention of venereal disease in black troops contributed to the problem of the soldiers becoming infected after entering the Army.[23]

The unpublished administrative history of the Navy that was written around the end of the war more clearly reveals the bias against African Americans. The volume on "The Negro in the Navy" discusses the "appallingly high" rate of venereal disease among "colored personnel," which "presented a borderline case between education and discipline." Although the policy of the Navy was to treat venereal disease cases as medical and not disciplinary problems, the "opinion was that it was necessary to resort to ultimate use of disciplinary measures more often regarding Negroes than whites." One disciplinary measure that was reportedly found to be effective with blacks was a diet of bread and water, "because of their heavy eating habits."[24]

An Army training film aimed at African American soldiers also reflects racial bias. Robert Eberwein has discussed how *Easy to Get* (1943) uses a voice-over by a white male to accompany most of the narrative scenes. The voice-over commentary tends to stress the ignorance of the black soldiers depicted, e.g., suggesting that a black soldier thought that "whores" were supposed to keep clean and should therefore be disease-free. While white soldiers were sometimes depicted in other military venereal disease films as being ignorant about certain aspects of sexual hygiene, Eberwein emphasizes that the comments about blacks in this film (sometimes supposedly actually reflecting the thoughts of the soldiers) "are pronounced by a white male" and "inflected with the ironic voice of white authority."[25]

Film historian Thomas Cripps criticized *Easy to Get*, which he called a "blundering" movie, for what he considered its portrayal of "black lasciviousness."[26] Sue Sun Yom, in her study of military venereal disease films, discussed how a particular dance scene in the film depicted "black sexual excess." African Americans are shown dancing to swing music. Although swing had become popular with whites in the 1940s, Yom

notes that black swing still "carried a whiff of impropriety and sexual endangerment."
She went on to say:

> In *Easy to Get*, the association between swing and black sexualization is established by
> rapid cuts between the alluring states of the black prostitute and the dancing couples
> in the middle of the juke joint's bar floor. . . . The impromptu swing demonstration
> highlights the physicality of black people and alludes to the possibility, in a wider
> cultural sense, of black contamination of white culture. . . . The set of shots immediately
> following the swing sequence makes the association between music and sexuality even
> more explicit. A long shot shows a debilitated black man lying in bed. "He was a hero
> in the last war," the narrator explains, "but he got syphilis from a whore overseas and
> did not take a medical leave to take care of it."[27]

An important World War II change in Army policy concerning venereal disease
was the removal of punishment for acquiring such a disease. It had been Army policy
since 1912 to withhold pay from soldiers with an injury or disease incurred while
they were not in the line of duty, and in 1926 Congress passed a statute requiring
loss of pay for soldiers contracting a venereal disease. The assumption behind this
action was that loss of pay would serve as a deterrent to exposure. During World War
II, however, a number of medical officers argued that this policy actually hindered
venereal disease control by encouraging soldiers to conceal their disease, and to treat
it with self-medication or by seeking the aid of a civilian physician who might not be
trained to deal with the disease. The soldier might then infect other civilian women,
who in turn could infect other soldiers. Others pointed out that the policy was unfair,
as men reacted differently to the disease and the treatment, and some soldiers would
be able to return to full-duty pay status sooner then others. On September 27, 1944,
Congress repealed the 1926 statute, and soldiers no longer lost pay as a result of
acquiring a venereal disease.[28]

Through various measures, the Army did manage to decrease the overall venereal
disease rate from 42.5 per 1,000 in 1940 to 25 per 1,000 in 1943. The incidence
for the entire duration of the war was 37 per 1,000, essentially equivalent to civilian
rates. Improved treatment regimens also cut the days lost to service because of these
diseases, even before the introduction of penicillin in 1943, which will be discussed
later in the chapter.[29]

MORALS AND MEDICINE: EDUCATING THE PUBLIC

As we have seen, the PHS under Surgeon General Thomas Parran had instituted
an extensive campaign of venereal disease education for the public beginning in 1936.
After the United States entered the war, this campaign intensified. Organizations such
as the ASHA, which had long been concerned with venereal disease education, also

contributed significantly to wartime efforts to inform the public about the venereal disease problem, but the focus here will be on the PHS effort. The education campaign utilized a variety of media, such as posters, publications, lectures, radio programs, and films to promote the goals of venereal disease control. The PHS also served as a cosponsor of the Venereal Disease Education Institute, established in Raleigh, North Carolina, in 1942, which provided a constant flow of educational materials for use in the campaign.[30]

The posters issued by the PHS, the military, the ASHA, and other organizations delivered a variety of antivenereal disease messages to both soldiers and civilians. Military posters focused on prophylaxis as well as abstinence, as noted above, but posters designed for civilian use generally avoided any mention of prophylaxis. These posters played on various emotions to promote behaviors that would reduce the risk of venereal disease. Patriotism in a country at war was an especially useful tool. Military posters, for example, showed caricatures of Hitler, Mussolini, and Tojo with messages such as "Fool the Axis—Use Prophylaxis." Venereal disease was often portrayed, usually in the form of a woman, as an ally of the Axis countries. One poster showed a woman with the face of death marching arm-in-arm with Hitler and Tojo, while the caption read "V.D.—Worst of the Three." Fear, guilt, faithfulness to wives and girlfriends, and other techniques were also employed in the poster campaign.[31]

As had always been the case, the sexual nature of the subject ensured that there would be tensions between a medical and a moralistic approach.[32] The PHS, as a government agency, had to walk a fine line with respect to venereal disease education. At times, the agency felt caught in the middle between competing and conflicting agendas. The Director of the DVD complained in 1944, for example:

Many physicians, health officers, and non-official organizations support and demand widespread, aggressive public education in the venereal diseases. When, following these demands, we attempt to conduct such education, the Public Health Service is attacked by groups who are opposed to the very concept of public education in this field.

. . . when we do nothing in this special aspect of the control program, other agencies begin promoting it. Sometimes their policies and objectives are not consonant with ours.[33]

The controversy over two of the films issued by the PHS during the war can serve to illustrate these tensions. The first of these films was *Know for Sure*, produced for the PHS in 1941 by the Research Council of the Academy of Motion Picture Arts as a part of its contribution to the war effort. The script incorporated information about syphilis provided by the PHS. The motion picture was designed to be shown to defense workers in airplane factories, ammunition plants, and other civil defense organizations. It was also used by other groups, including the military. It was clearly meant to be shown to male workers, but a version of the film omitting the scenes involving male genitalia and the use of prophylactics was later produced for mixed audiences. Although no cast credits were given, a number of Hollywood actors donated their services to appear in the film, including J. Carrol Naish, Tim Holt, Samuel Hinds, and Ward Bond. African American actress Hattie McDaniel also appeared in the film, playing a role that combined stereotypes of black women, namely an "Aunt Jemima" type who worked as a maid in a brothel.

The film begins with the story of Tony, a stereotypical Italian immigrant with an accent and an emotional temperament. He is very excited about the impending birth of his first child, but is devastated when the baby is born dead, the victim of congenital syphilis passed on by Tony to his wife. The distraught Tony threatens to kill himself, but the doctor calms him down and explains that he and his wife can be cured and can have children in the future. The film then depicts several other brief vignettes dealing with men who contracted syphilis through contact with prostitutes or "pick-ups," and one involving a syphilitic man who is robbed of his money and his health by a quack doctor. Although the film warns of the dangers of casual sex, it is not overly moralistic in its tone. The motion picture devotes substantial attention to methods for minimizing the risks of contracting venereal disease, including explicit visual demonstrations of how to use a condom and how to properly cleanse the genitals after sex. The film also emphasizes the importance of seeking qualified medical attention in cases of suspected infection and notes that one can only "know for sure" whether he has the disease by a blood test. Another key message of the film is that syphilis is curable with the proper medical attention.[34]

The PHS made a conscious decision to make prophylaxis an essential message of this film. Perhaps the urgency of war convinced Parran and other leaders at PHS that they needed to more explicitly discuss the use of condoms and other prophylactic methods in contrast to their earlier relative avoidance of the subject. One PHS officer referred to *Know for Sure* specifically as "the prophylaxis film" in a letter. Another PHS officer stated not long after the film came out that there was no question in his mind that considerable emphasis must be given to prophylaxis in any PHS venereal disease motion pictures. The Service was well aware that the decision to focus the film so much on prophylaxis would be controversial. In an effort to minimize this criticism, the PHS decided to distribute the film mainly through local health agencies. Even the copies to be distributed directly by the PHS would only be loaned on the endorsement of a local health agency. As a PHS officer explained in a letter to Vonderlehr:

> The purpose of this arrangement is to forestall unnecessary criticism—which is sure to fall on any motion picture treating prophylaxis. Also, when the film is used in restricted groups under proper supervision, its effects can be supplemented from the local authorities and the subject matter better related to local situations.[35]

These precautions, however, by no means eliminated all criticism of the film. Even Dr. Walter Clarke, director of the ASHA, complained to Vonderlehr about the

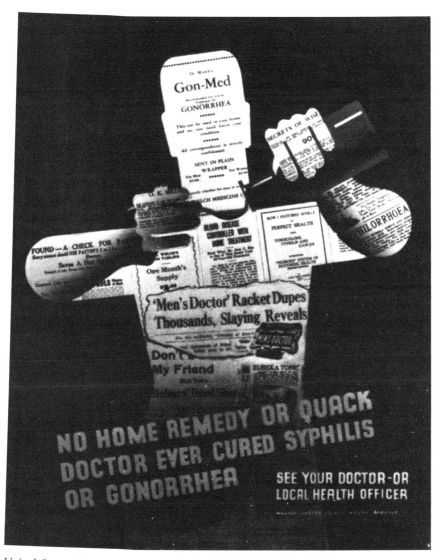

United States Public Health Service poster of the 1940s warning against relying on quack doctors and remedies to treat venereal disease [Courtesy of the National Library of Medicine].

depiction of prophylactic methods in the film. In reply, Vonderlehr wrote that the belief of the PHS "was and still is that a certain number of men are going to find and use opportunities for extramarital sex relations no matter what happens," and that preventing infection was an important part of the agency's job. In his view, "Teaching men how to protect themselves from venereal disease does not imply that we condone sexual promiscuity no more than teaching soldiers how to protect themselves against poison gas proves that the Army wishes to encourage the use of such gas by the enemy."

Clarke also voiced the view that the film, although it did point to prostitution as a major source of infection, should have devoted more attention to the subject on moral grounds. Vonderlehr countered that he favored the repression of prostitution, but that in his capacity as a public health official he distinguished between the moral and medical aspects of the problem. He concluded, "If all men invariably protected themselves, then, from a public health standpoint, prostitution unlimited would not concern us as health officers, even though we might object to it on other grounds."[36]

The executive officer of the Montana State Board of Health raised a concern about whether the film might "encourage sex immorality and birth control." PHS officer E. R. Coffey responded that the PHS believed the need for enlightenment on methods of preventing venereal disease outweighed other considerations and that he was confident that those who saw the motion picture would understand that the objective was not to encourage immorality but to prevent the spread of disease. The venereal disease subcommittee of the Philadelphia Defense Council also protested to the PHS about the film and suggested that the section on prophylaxis be removed. Raymond Vonderlehr replied that prophylaxis was a primary educational message of the film, and noted that the PHS had already received a large number of favorable responses to the film. *Know for Sure* was indeed well received by many, including the Army, the Navy, and the American Public Health Association. In response to a comment that the film should have devoted more attention to continence, another PHS officer writing in 1944 stated that when *Know for Sure* was made, there were numerous other films available that stressed continence. Thus the PHS had decided to emphasize neglected aspects of the subject, such as prophylaxis, the dangers of quack treatment, and the importance of early diagnosis and treatment.[37]

The PHS encountered further controversy with respect to another motion picture, *To the People of the United States*, released in 1944. It was produced by Walter Wanger Productions, which was affiliated with Universal Studios, in conjunction with the PHS and the California Health Department. Walter Wanger offered to donate his services to make the film, and he arranged for various actors, writers, and technician to do the same as a Hollywood contribution to the war effort. Wanger envisioned that the film would be shown in theaters nationwide as a short, along with the usual double feature. PHS leaders thought this was a wonderful opportunity to obtain a film that would be suitable for widespread viewing in motion picture theaters. Such a film, of course, would have to be suitable for mixed gender audiences and could not contain any sexually explicit material if it had any hope of being accepted by theater managers. It would also have to have enough dramatic interest to have some entertainment as well as educational value.[38]

To the People of the United States was completed by about the end of 1943. Hollywood star Jean Hersholt donated his services to play the protagonist, an army doctor. Other actors who participated in the film included Noah Beery, Jr., and Robert Mitchum. The movie begins with introductory statements by Army Surgeon General

Norman Kirk and PHS Surgeon General Thomas Parran. It then moves to a scene of American bombers taking off from an airfield. A disappointed pilot, grounded because he has syphilis, watches the planes leave. He is concerned that he will never fly again, but the doctor played by Hersholt explains that the disease is treatable and the pilot can be cured. Much of the rest of the film is devoted to a comparison of syphilis rates and attitudes toward the disease in the United States versus Scandinavian countries. The openness in talking about venereal disease in Scandinavia, much admired by Parran, is contrasted with the American practice of not discussing the problem in public. Americans are encouraged to confront the disease openly. Except for a final statement by Parran, the film ends with scenes of farmers, factory workers, soldiers, athletes, Boy Scouts, and schoolchildren at work and play, while Hersholt's voice is heard above the stirring music proclaiming:

> The children who follow us must inherit health—and freedom—and happiness. . . . The Scourge of Disease must be wiped from the land, and then there will be a new day ahead. . . . A day without insidious, lurking evil sicknesses—a day without a useless hypocritical attitude which refuses to name a germ—yet permits the horrible devastation caused by it. . . . Syphilis! Say it . . . Learn about it! Have a blood test to make sure you haven't got it! And, working together, we'll stamp it out. . . . [39]

The PHS, which had reviewed and approved the script, was basically pleased with the final product. Parran declared that the film would be "extremely valuable for use in an intensified national program of public education and information which will begin early in the new year." He was negotiating with the Office of War Information (OWI) to arrange for national commercial theater distribution. Since the film was designed for widespread viewing by the general public, it did not contain any graphic scenes explicitly depicting sexual organs or the disease, and it avoided controversial subjects such as prostitution and prophylaxis. Parran must have assumed that this film was not likely to provoke the type of criticism that *Know for Sure* had. Stanton Griffis, chief of the OWI's Bureau of Motion Pictures, viewed the film and recommended that it be accepted as part of the OWI program. He expressed the view that the film was "brilliantly made" and did not see anything in it "that could offend man, woman or child, except a prude still wandering in the haze of a social viewpoint of bygone days."[40]

In spite of the confidence of Parran and Griffis that the film should not offend anyone, it ran into trouble even before its release. In March, the Legion of Decency, established by the Catholic Church to evaluate whether or not films were "morally objectionable," reviewed the film and protested against it to the OWI and the PHS. While admitting that venereal disease was a threat to the war effort, the Legion did not believe that movie theaters were an appropriate venue for dealing with the problem. Representatives of the PHS and the ASHA met with Legion officials to discuss their objections to the motion picture. In the 1930s, Hollywood had instituted the Motion Picture Code to establish moral guidelines for theatrical films, and one of the strictures of the Code was against films on sex hygiene and venereal disease. Although *To the People of the United States* was not a commercial film, the Legion believed that it should follow the Code if it was intended for release in theaters. Representatives of the Legion also expressed concern that such a film would "pave the way for a flood of pictures by producers who do not hesitate to avail themselves of every opportunity for lurid and pornographic material for financial gain." Finally, they were unhappy that the film failed "to stress the fact that promiscuity is the principal cause for the spread of venereal disease." Admitting that the film presented its subject matter in "an essentially dignified and restrained" manner, the Legion still asked the PHS not to sponsor it for theatrical release.[41]

Parran turned for advice on this situation to the PHS Advisory Committee on Public Education for the Prevention of Venereal Diseases, composed of clergymen, health professionals, and teachers. The Committee advised the Surgeon General that in their view, given the opposition that had been voiced, it would not be wise for the PHS to sponsor theatrical release of the film. They were concerned that such an action "might endanger the whole program of venereal disease education and might even have harmful effects on other vital and important public health activities throughout the nation." The Committee did suggest, however, that with minor changes the film would be suitable for controlled distribution through state and local health departments, voluntary health agencies, and similar organizations. They recommended in particular that "some attention be given to the influence of moral standards on the spread of disease" because if no reference was made to moral issues, it might appear to some that the PHS was "condoning sexual promiscuity."[42]

Parran decided to accept the advisory group's recommendations. The film would receive only limited distribution through health agencies and similar organizations, and would not be released in theaters. The Surgeon General also bowed to concerns that there was no reference to moral issues in *To the People of the United States* by revising his brief speech at the end of the film. His new closing words emphasized promiscuity as a major cause of venereal disease and gave credit to various groups combating this problem.

> Here, we have told only part of the story of venereal disease control. Untold is the fine work our churches, schools, and social agencies are doing to prevent the promiscuity which spreads infection. It is important to remember that the only sure way to avoid infection is to avoid exposure.[43]

Out of a concern about the damage that a controversy over the film might inflict on the PHS venereal disease campaign and other programs, Parran elected to yield to religious and social pressures on this issue. He recognized that the film would not be seen by as many people if it were not shown in commercial theaters, but he accepted the compromise position of limited distribution to appease the Legion of Decency and other critics. Parran had already shown his willingness to tackle controversial issues, but he was enough of a politician to know when it would be wise to give ground.

The reaction to these two films provides examples of the controversies that the PHS and other agencies had to contend with in their venereal disease education campaigns. Criticism, however, was not limited to motion pictures. For example, the PHS ran afoul of the Catholic Church again in 1944 in connection with a brochure that had been developed by the Service as a part of its education campaign. The PHS brochure was being distributed by the War Advertising Council, a nonprofit organization of advertising executives, to national advertisers, advertising agencies, and newspapers in the hopes that they would run public service announcements using illustrated copy provided in the brochure. Catholic organizations such as the Catholic War Veterans and the Knights of Columbus opposed the distribution of the brochure, characterizing the publication as "indecent, repulsive, and un-American," and also criticizing it for its "offensive frankness." Yielding to this pressure, the Council withdrew its support of the PHS venereal disease campaign.[44]

In spite of the fact that *Know for Sure*, released in 1943 and intended for a limited audience, had emphasized prophylaxis, it is clear that the PHS remained cautious about discussing the subject in its campaign. It was not mentioned at all, for example, in the 1944 *To the People of the United States*, which originally had been targeted for a broader audience. In addition, in a document providing guidance to the media on presenting venereal disease information to the public issued by the PHS and the OWI in January 1944, the list of "Don'ts" included the following item: "Don't associate the education program, directly or indirectly, with mechanical prophylaxis or contraceptive methods."[45]

Some of the PHS educational materials were aimed at specific segments of the population, such as women or African Americans. Sometimes essentially the same poster was produced in both "black" and "white" versions (i.e., depicting either African Americans or whites, but using the same message). In other cases, the materials were completely different. To my knowledge, the PHS did not produce a motion picture film specifically for blacks during World War II, and it was not until late in the war that it issued a film aimed at female audiences, *A Message to Women* (1945). Produced for the PHS and the Tennessee Department of Public Health by Hugh Harmon Productions, *A Message to Women* was a twenty-minute color film employing professional actors. It told the story of Peggy Parker, a young, single woman who learns from her doctor that she has gonorrhea. The doctor chastises Peggy's mother for not providing her with appropriate information about sex and venereal disease. The rest of the film focuses on Mrs. Parker's attendance at meetings of her club and a hygiene association where the dangers of venereal disease are discussed.

The film was designed to be shown to women's organizations, service clubs, and older teenage girls. An important part of its message was that venereal disease strikes without regard to family position or background. "Respectable" girls and their mothers should not assume that venereal disease is not a problem that they need worry about. Cinema historian Robert Eberwein has pointed out that *A Message for Women* is one of the few films of the period in which a woman infected with a venereal disease was not depicted as a prostitute or a so-called pick-up. There is no discussion in the film of prophylactic measures such as condoms. The only form of prevention promoted is abstinence. As Eberwein has noted, the film warns women "that the only way to remain free of venereal disease is to avoid sex outside of marriage."[46]

PROSTITUTION AND PROMISCUITY

As was the case in the past, women (especially prostitutes and those considered promiscuous) received a substantial portion of the blame in the World War II venereal disease campaign. Posters aimed at soldiers or male civilians warned men about getting sexually involved with prostitutes or "good-time girls." Such women were considered to invariably be carriers of syphilis or gonorrhea. When personified, venereal disease was always portrayed as a woman in these posters, as in the example cited above of the female figure with the face of death marching arm-in-arm with Hitler and Tojo. Other posters depicted seductive but "disreputable-looking" women, often with a cigarette dangling from the mouth, described as "a bag of trouble" or a "juke joint sniper." It was not just the woman who was or looked like a prostitute, however, that posed a danger. Other posters depicted "girl-next-door" types with warnings such as "She may look clean—but . . ."[47]

The federal government, as it had in World War I, developed mechanisms for trying to keep the areas surrounding military camps free of prostitutes. The May Act, discussed above, was one such measure. The ASHA once again sent its investigators into the field to report on prostitution and vice in American cities. The Secretary of War wrote to all state governors requesting their cooperation in keeping the areas around the camps free of commercial prostitution. In late 1941, a new agency, the Social Protection Division (SPD), was created within the Federal Security Agency to help enforce the provisions against prostitution.[48]

Part of the reason for creating such a unit, whose chief task was described as promoting "the reduction of venereal disease through the repression of commercialized prostitution," was noted in a statement that defined the relationship of the SPD to the PHS, both of which were housed in the Federal Security Agency. This document explained that the PHS, although it was charged with controlling venereal disease, preferred "not to carry the responsibility for bringing pressure upon law enforcement officials" who were not diligent in their repression of prostitution. The statement also

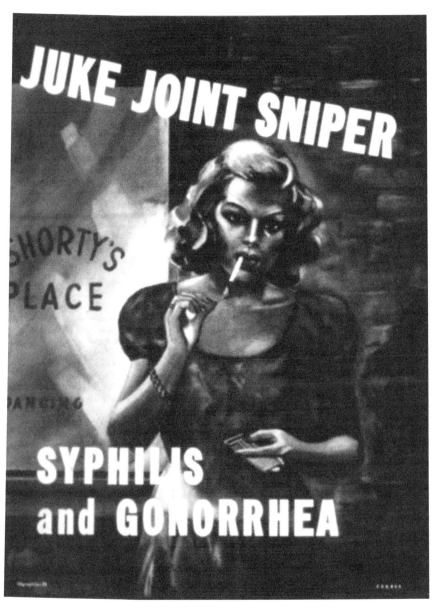

World War II American poster equating a prostitute, presumed to be a carrier of venereal disease, with an enemy sniper [Courtesy of the National Library of Medicine].

emphasized the view that the prostitute was "the chief agent for the spread of venereal disease."[49]

The Surgeon General and the PHS agreed that prostitution was an important source of venereal disease and supported its repression. When a PHS physician stationed in Puerto Rico suggested in 1942 that registration of prostitutes might be a good idea, Parran reprimanded him. Noting that he understood that the physician probably looked upon registration as a means of controlling the disease, Parran nevertheless informed him that such a system would be out of line with federal policy. The practical result, Parran pointed out, "would seem to be an official toleration of commercialized prostitution." Any system other than rigid repression of prostitution, he added, would be contrary to PHS policy, to which the doctor in question had to conform. However, the PHS obviously preferred to concern itself with the medical aspects of the problem, and not to become involved with the policing of prostitution.[50]

To head the new SPD, the government selected Eliot Ness, who had achieved fame (and later almost mythic status thanks to movies and television) as a Prohibition agent. His team of Prohibition agents had been dubbed by a Chicago newspaper reporter "The Untouchables" because they could not be bought. Ness helped to compile the evidence that convicted Al Capone on income tax evasion charges in 1931. Late in 1935 he became Director of Public Safety for the city of Cleveland, where he became known for cracking down on vice and organized crime. When the SPD was formed, Ness also began serving as a consultant to the new agency. He was appointed director of the SPD in the spring of 1942. It is ironic that his new job involved combating venereal disease, as his old nemesis Al Capone was by then suffering from syphilitic dementia.[51]

Ness labeled venereal disease "military saboteur number one," and spent much of his time on the job at military bases, where he lectured and distributed literature. He also worked with local law enforcement officials to ensure their cooperation in the effort to eliminate prostitution in areas near military installations. He threatened to revoke the licenses of bars, taxi drivers, and others who were involved in providing prostitutes to soldiers. Ness biographer Paul Heimel described one incident where Ness was speaking in Peoria, Illinois, when a group of prostitutes and their supporters held a protest, "harassing the audience and displaying signs decrying Ness's actions as an affront to their personal liberties."[52]

At a national conference in 1943, Ness reported on the work of the SPD, which by then had a staff of ten in the Washington office and some thirty-eight in the field. He proclaimed that during the time the SPD had been in existence, known houses of prostitution and "red-light districts" had been closed in 662 cities and towns. Furthermore, he announced, the Division had enlisted the cooperation of organizations and private enterprises in attacking clandestine prostitution and promiscuity in general. He also indicated that he was planning to do more to enlist the help of black leaders in dealing with prostitution in African American neighborhoods. He hoped in this manner to combat charges that police action against brothels in these neighborhoods, which often housed both black and white prostitutes, represented racial persecution. Overall, he stated, his goal was "a free America that will be physically healthy, mentally alert and morally sound."[53]

As Allan Brandt has pointed out, the attention of the military and the SPD soon came to focus not only on prostitutes, but also on any woman who was considered promiscuous or of loose morals. Those responsible for protecting the troops against venereal disease came to see these women as an even greater threat to the war effort than "professional" prostitutes. Closing the "red light districts" did not solve the venereal disease problem, and increasingly physicians reported that prostitutes constituted only a minority of the sexual contacts of soldiers. One journalist made the possibly exaggerated claim (as quoted by Brandt) that "[f]ully 90 percent of the Army's cases in this country are traceable to amateur girls—teenagers and older women—popularly known as 'khaki-wackies,' 'victory girls,' and 'good-time Charlottes.'"[54]

This view of course reflected the continued double standard in America with respect to sexuality. As Brandt has stated:

> Indeed, the word "promiscuous" was firmly anchored to "girl"—a promiscuous man was, by definition, an oxymoron. Women in this view, were the keepers of sexual mores—their indiscretion led to a deterioration of morals. "They" infected the soldiers; in this view, venereal disease could only be transmitted in one direction. Therefore, as sexual mores did in fact change, the burden of this transformation came to be placed upon women.[55]

Military and public health leaders did not care whether these women were prostitutes or "victory girls"—all were seen as threats to servicemen and essential war workers. Public officials were ready and willing to take extreme measures to counter this perceived menace, including quarantining women with venereal disease, leading to the creation of venereal disease rapid treatment centers.

QUARANTINING WOMEN: VENEREAL DISEASE RAPID TREATMENT CENTERS

As the war progressed, the demand on existing clinic and hospital facilities for the treatment of venereal disease increased, creating pressure for new facilities. In addition, jails became overcrowded since efforts to crack down on prostitution generally entailed subjecting the arrested women to mandatory venereal examinations, and treating them under detention if they were infected. As in World War I, public officials were concerned that prostitutes would not comply with the treatment regimen if not forced to. The newly developed rapid treatment methods, discussed in the last chapter, seemed to offer more promise in terms of treating these women in a short period of time under supervision as in-patients in a hospital or clinic. Finally, some public health officials believed that it was necessary to provide more than medical treatment to prostitutes and "loose women." They believed that it was also important to "redirect" these women towards "higher" morals and, in the case of prostitutes, a new occupation.[56]

These factors led to the development of a plan to establish a series of rapid treatment centers, which were described as "a direct and realistic effort to combat the venereal diseases as a wartime threat to our national security."[57] By late 1942, the PHS was developing plans, in conjunction with the Federal Works Agency and the Office of Defense Health and Welfare Services, for hospital facilities "to provide care for prostitutes and other promiscuous females who have a venereal disease."[58] Originally the proposal was that the PHS would operate these hospitals as a temporary measure, and then turn them over to state department of health. Eventually it was decided, however, that it would be better to have state or local authorities operate such quarantine hospitals from the beginning, with the PHS operating such a facility only when it was considered a necessity in a given area and the state health department refused to assume the responsibility.[59]

Funding for the construction, maintenance, and operation of the hospitals was provided to the states by the federal government under the Lanham Acts of 1941. These two bills appropriated funds for defense housing and for community facilities in war areas. If the appropriate war agencies certified the defense need of a project, it was eligible for funding under the Lanham Acts. The venereal disease quarantine hospitals were considered to be necessary from a defense point of view. Since these funds could not be used for the medical care of the patients, the PHS provided monies for this purpose to the states under the Venereal Disease Control Act. In addition, the PHS agreed to provide each hospital, in so far as possible, with a medical officer in charge, a head nurse, a record analyst, and several psychiatrists.[60]

It is clear that these facilities were originally intended for prostitutes, and probably so-called promiscuous women as well, although later in the war some also began to admit men. The main reason for creating them was as an emergency wartime measure, to protect the troops and civilian war workers against venereal disease. The first time that the entry "Rapid Treatment Centers" appeared in the index of the PHS journal *Venereal Disease Information* in 1943, for example, it reads as follows: "Rapid treatment centers *See* Prostitutes, rapid treatment of." Correspondence of the period also makes clear the initial purpose of the centers. In one letter in 1942, for example, Raymond Vonderlehr of the PHS referred to them as "detention centers to provide treatment for prostitutes infected with a venereal disease." The quotation above about these facilities providing for the care of "prostitutes and other promiscuous females" with a venereal disease is from a 1943 letter written by Surgeon General Parran. In another 1942 letter, the assistant chief of the DVD referred to quarantine hospital facilities to be used in caring for prostitutes.[61]

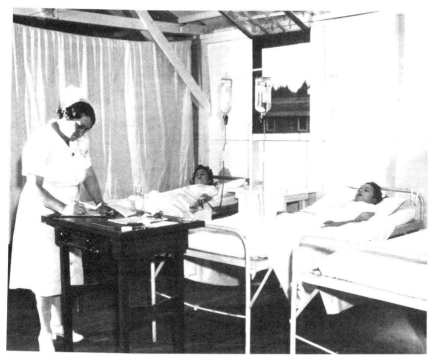

Nurse attending female patients in a World War II American venereal disease rapid treatment center [Courtesy of the National Library of Medicine].

A number of these hospitals, or rapid treatment centers, were established in former work camps used by the Civilian Conservation Corps (CCC), the Depression-era agency created by the federal government to provide employment for jobless young men. The suggestion to use these camps apparently came from Eliot Ness. The Federal Security Agency arranged for the transfer of many of these former CCC camps to state health department for use as rapid treatment centers. In addition, remodeled small hotels, sanatoria, and hospital buildings, as well as special wards in general hospitals, were also used for this purpose. Over twenty centers were established during the first year of the program in 1943, and by 1947 there were forty-seven of these facilities throughout the United States, many of them located near Army or Navy training facilities or important war-industry cities. The capacities of these hospitals varied greatly, from perhaps a couple of dozen to over 300 patients.[62]

Treatment largely involved the arsenic-bismuth rapid therapy for syphilis and sulfa drug therapy for gonorrhea discussed in the previous chapter, although fever and heat therapy were also sometimes employed. When penicillin became available late in the war, it was used where possible in the centers. Depending upon the method employed, complete treatment could take from days to weeks. Patients were also kept at the center under observation for a period of about four to eight weeks after treatment to ensure that the therapy had actually been successful. In addition, the centers frequently provided some vocational training for patients. The PHS indicated that it expected that the maximum stay would not exceed ten weeks.[63]

The quarantining of women with venereal disease was a repetition of what had happened in World War I. Once again women were made to bear the brunt of the blame for the spread of venereal disease. There was no similar system of quarantine hospitals established for infected men. Although these facilities were sometimes referred to as quarantine hospitals for prostitutes, it is clear that any infected woman who was deemed a threat to the war effort could be confined in a rapid treatment center and made to undergo therapy.

An article in the April 10, 1943 issue of *Collier's Magazine* entitled "The War Against Syphilis" provided a vivid portrayal of how women were detained at the Leesville Quarantine Hospital. The facility was located in Leesville, Louisiana, near Camp Polk, an army training facility. The author of the article, J. D. Ratcliff, describes the quarantine hospital as "a camp for women of easy virtue." All of the inmates, he added, had a venereal disease, and would be treated and cured before being released. Ratcliff justified the need for the hospital by explaining that simply fining such women and putting them in jail for a few days did nothing to halt the spread of venereal disease. He noted that, "It was like fining a typhoid carrier and telling her to carry no more typhoid." One wonders whether he had in mind the famous case of "Typhoid Mary" (Mary Mallon), the Irish-American cook who was a healthy carrier of typhoid disease in early twentieth-century America and was held in quarantine for years by New York public health officials. In fact, in 1940, the *Journal of Social Hygiene* had compared "Typhoid Mary" to "Spirochete Annie."[64]

The head of venereal disease work for the Louisiana State Board of Health was able to utilize state legislation that permitted the isolation of people with communicable diseases as a basis for detaining the women, as was true in most states. In his article, Ratcliff described how the women to be detained were identified:

> When Army doctors discover a soldier has a venereal disease, he is questioned at length. Lists of his contacts are made, and the girls are rounded up for a check. If blood tests show they have syphilis or if there is evidence of gonorrhea, they are taken to the hospital immediately.
>
> The health men of the parish (county) pick up diseased girls in their routine examination of food handlers. State police meet incoming buses. Unescorted girls who get off are questioned. If they are coming to meet husbands who are in the Army, or if they have other legitimate business, the troopers assist them. But if they give unsatisfactory answers, they are politely informed that they must undergo examination.[65]

Historian Marilyn Hegarty, who has examined a study of the Leesville facility, reported that "suspect women" could be arrested on a variety of charges, such as vagrancy and loitering, or even "on suspicion." One married woman was picked up when she stopped to eat lunch alone on her way home from her job as a waitress (an occupation that occasioned suspicion). She was charged with vagrancy and pressured to commit herself voluntarily to the quarantine hospital. However, she tested negative for venereal disease. Another woman was picked up for drunkenness. Although she listed no occupation on her intake from, a social worker typed in "prostitute." She may have been suspect because she was known to belong to a local commune, where it was believed that sexual relations were "easy." Many of the residents of the commune received relief, and were perceived as problems by the police. In addition, the detained woman's mother worked at a "disreputable place," and therefore she and her daughters were viewed as "probably delinquent."[66]

Ratcliff estimated, although who knows on what basis, that probably no more than 5 percent of the women who were picked up were professional prostitutes. The rest, he said, were young girls "caught up by the excitement of war" who had left home seeking adventure. Such amateurs, he argued, were more dangerous than professionals, because they had less knowledge about how to care for themselves (presumably he meant how to protect themselves against venereal disease). Although he indicated that the women could come from the "whole scale" of social backgrounds, his biases with respect to women who were black and/or poor are obvious. At the top, he noted, were college women who have had "a moral smash-up." At the bottom were "14-year old Negro girls from share-cropper homes, with no particular desire in life beyond owning a pair of yellow rayon slacks and a pair of spike-heeled shoes."[67] This contempt is also reflected in his comment about the camp followers who came to Leesville, "Girls who had been raised in one-room swamp cabins—and for whom sex held no sweet mysteries—moved to town. Here was their chance to get the fancy raiment in mail-order catalogues."[68]

Ratcliff's concern about the uncontrolled sexuality of young women whom he viewed as delinquent was shared by many social welfare and public health workers as well. One PHS officer, in an article about the rapid treatment centers, wrote of the "immature teen-age girls who have left their farm homes or their little towns" in search of defense jobs or following boyhood sweethearts. To him, it was obvious that throwing together young, immature girls with men living away from home could have only one result, "sexual delinquency." The war situation had led to "increased numbers of young girls who brazenly parade from one honky-tonk to another and who end up tragically infected in our offices or clinics." Although admitting that the boy friends of these girls were also delinquents, it is clear that his emphasis was on controlling the sexuality of the young women and in making sure that they complied with the treatment regimen. Note the tone of the following quotation from this article and the number of times that the word "control" is used.

[A]ll of us have had some bitter experiences with these girls. Time and again medical personnel would give these young girls sulfathiazole pills to cure them of gonorrhea and they would go home, take five or six, become a bit nauseated and throw the rest in the wastebasket. It would be a week or two weeks before this failure to take treatment would be discovered and in the meantime the girl was continuing her promiscuous activity. . . . We all began to realize we needed a greater element of *control* over these girls. We needed to remove them from the community and *control* them so that they could not continue their promiscuous activity. We needed to *control* them so that we could be absolutely sure that they received every bit of the treatment that they so badly needed. [italics mine][69]

Another article by a San Francisco public health official and the president of the ASHA emphasized that "the promiscuous girl has come to be considered the major source of venereal infection." The authors speculated that this problem would only become worse in the future because of the "the lowering of moral conduct and the loosening of old controls and safeguards." They reflected with seeming nostalgia that just a few decades earlier "a promiscuous woman would find her door painted with tar as the sign of disapproval of her amoral behavior."[70] A PHS physician who conducted a study of some 300 women in a rapid treatment center in St. Louis claimed that a considerable number of them admitted to being indiscriminate in their choice of male companions. Though they were promiscuous, the doctor noted, they resented any inference that they were prostitutes. In his view, their low ethical standards must stem from either "a lack of moral consciousness" (i.e., amoral behavior) or an aggressive response of the individual, expressed through sexual delinquency, toward the community.[71] The sexual behavior of so-called promiscuous women was repeatedly explained by health and social workers as being caused by such factors as a broken home, hypersexuality, mental deficiency, or mental illness. Clearly these largely middle-class professionals could not understand or accept sexual mores that differed from their own, at least in women.[72]

As indicated above, admittance to a rapid treatment center was not always on a voluntary basis, nor were patients necessarily free to leave of their own accord. Many were confined to the centers under state laws involving the control of communicable diseases, i.e., they were considered to be quarantined. Not only were they detained in these facilities, but they were required to accept treatment until they had been cured of the disease. A guide to the operation of the centers developed by the PHS commented as follows on the admission and release of patients:

At the discretion of the State Health Officer, admission to Rapid Treatment Centers may be on a voluntary or involuntary basis. In either case persons suspected of having, known to have had, or who have been under observation for a venereal disease may be committed. Involuntary admissions should result principally from commitments under quarantine laws. Normal patients will be released after a reasonable observation period (approximately four to eight weeks) following completion of treatment. Release of patients admitted involuntarily should be at the discretion of the State Health Officer or his deputy.[73]

Police and health officials did not hesitate to use the powers at their command to detain infected women. However, it may not have always been necessary to actually forcibly quarantine a patient as there were other ways of exerting pressure. A PHS report made the point that sometimes the threat of court action was all that was necessary to induce an uncooperative patient to undergo treatment. Various officials expressed the hope that over time the majority of admissions would become voluntary.[74]

In addition to medical treatment, many of the centers tried to utilize some of the time that the women were quarantined to give them at least minimal vocational training, although the extent of such training varied from center to center. The purpose was to encourage the women to find gainful employment when they were released from the hospital, instead of going back to prostitution if that had been their means of support. As one PHS physician wrote in 1943, "The object of the program is to direct these girls, after they are physically fit, to war industries in order to raise their economic status so as to eliminate their turning to prostitution to supplement their low incomes." In fact, Surgeon General Parran himself had suggested in 1942 that prostitutes, after being cured of VD, be trained for jobs in war industries. The women were also often responsible for some of the work involved in the operation of the center, such as cooking, sewing, cleaning, and waiting on tables. This work was also often considered to be training. The PHS guide for the centers advocated paying the patients for such work, but it is not clear whether or not this was done as a general practice. As penicillin became more available, treatment regimes were considerably shortened and patients released earlier, making it more difficult to provide any vocational training.[75]

The PHS also made psychiatric and counseling services available to the centers, since, in the words of the PHS guide, "many of the patients are likely to have emotional and adjustment difficulties." One PHS doctor stated that it was a "known fact" that many of the "girls" were not employable because of mental deficiency or emotional disturbance. A treatise on counseling in the rapid treatment centers by a PHS occupational specialist pointed out, however, that the centers had neither the time nor the expertise to provide comprehensive social service counseling. The main objective of the PHS was to ensure that none of the patients were "turned loose without defense against the social problem that may in part have been responsible for the original infection." The PHS had to rely extensively on resources in the community to provide the additional assistance required to "render the patient capable of participating fully in the normal life of today."[76]

In addition, the rapid treatment centers were encouraged to provide recreational opportunities for the patients, such as dancing and singing. On this subject, the PHS guide stated that adequate facilities and opportunities for "wholesome recreation" would aid in creating a cooperative attitude, as well as in keeping the patient physically fit. Games, craft classes, informal dramatics and special holiday parties were among the recommended activities.[77] One case worker described a typical day at the Lebanon, Pennsylvania, quarantine facility, which apparently did not provide vocational training beyond domestic skills, as follows:

> While the girls are at the hospital they assist with the work, with cleaning and sewing, waiting on tables, kitchen work, etc. They rise at 7 o'clock in the morning, eat breakfast, receive medication and they do the morning cleaning and laundry work. They have their lunch at noon, and after lunch, they take short walks on the grounds and are allowed recreation. From 2 to 4 p.m. is their rest period, and from 4 to 6 they sew, making uniforms and bandages for the hospital. After dinner, with dishes washed and everything in order, they have entertainment, such as games, dancing, and singing. Girls who smoke are allowed five cigarettes a day. There is a small commissary where the girls may buy candy, cosmetics, cigarettes, writing paper. All holidays and anniversaries are celebrated by having parties. Visitors are not allowed, but the girls may write letters.[78]

Although African American and white patients were often quarantined in the same hospitals, they were apparently generally segregated with respect to their living quarters. Race relations between patients, or between patients and staff, were not always smooth. Reports from centers in Florida, for example, referred to difficulties and disturbances between whites and blacks, and even made a point in describing one situation involving white patients to specify that it was not in this case a "white versus colored riot." Another report from a Florida facility described an "uprising" that began as a result of an argument between one of the African American patients and a male carpenter employed at the hospital. When the woman refused to obey an order from the carpenter, he slapped her. After the incident, the black patients, according to the report, "began to assemble and howl." The patient was admonished for failing to follow a lawful order, but the carpenter was suspended pending an investigation because rough handling of the patients was forbidden. He immediately quit in anger. Further disturbances, however, broke out later in the day, including a battle between black and white patients at the canteen. The report also stated: "The colored patients then paraded the hospital area abusing with utmost profanity the matrons and workers on the area. Assemblies were broken up many times, but race hatred was demonstrated in many ways." The sheriff was called in and brought police officers with him because he was reportedly concerned that "anything could happen with colored women in that frame of mind."[79]

This last comment reflects of course the continuing racial bias and condescension of many whites toward African Americans. For example, a 1947 thesis on administrative problems in rapid treatment centers, written by a physician as a requirement for his Master of Public Health degree, is rife with stereotypical negative views of blacks. The document noted that many patients were "uneducated plantation negroes inherently suspicious of everyone in the white race not associated with the plantation." It went on to state that some of the blacks were believers in voodoo and that superstitions are "deeply rooted into the lives of the southern negro, and reasoning is of no avail." The author described an incident, which he termed "ludicrous," where about fifty black women fled a ward one night after supposedly seeing a ghost. In another section of the dissertation, the author claimed that black patients were in the habit of saying "yes, mam," whether or not they understood a request. He also expressed the views that the black patients knew syphilis only as "bad blood" and had no understanding of its venereal connection, and that a large number of them had common law spouses (sometimes several). White patients were not singled out for any specific criticisms.[80]

Marilyn Hegarty has pointed out that officials of the SPD (and of other government agencies), although admitting that factors such as low economic status and inferior educational and health care systems played a role in the higher venereal disease rate of blacks, tended to view African Americans as being apathetic concerning venereal disease. White officials generally ignored the long history of efforts to combat venereal disease in African American communities. They also dismissed attempts by black leaders to question the statistics on venereal disease. In addition, according to Hegarty, they commonly accepted the "stereotype of hypersexuality as characteristic of black persons, especially black women."[81]

The stereotyping of African Americans (and also women) is also reflected in a film on the centers produced by the Department of Agriculture for the PHS in 1944. Entitled simply *Venereal Disease Rapid Treatment Center*, the film is ten minutes in length and was evidently made to explain and justify the facilities. The motion picture emphasizes that these centers are hospitals, and that the patients are far better off in these facilities than in the squalid jails found in many areas. In a segment of the film dealing with recreational activities at the center depicted, which was only for females, white patients are shown putting on a musical show. Black patients, on the other hand, are shown jitterbugging, while the narrator exclaims, "The Negro patients enjoy dancing—and how!"[82]

The PHS took pains to stress, as in the film about the rapid treatment centers, that these centers were hospitals, similar to other types of quarantine hospitals, and not prisons. On one occasion, Raymond Vonderlehr complained to a colleague about a center that was surrounded by high fences with locked gates and used barbed wire charged with electricity. In addition, the facility contained many women with criminal charges against them. Vonderlehr worried that these features gave the center "the characteristic of a penal institution, rather than a medical center with a rehabilitation program." As the centers began to receive more patients who were viewed as women gone astray, rather than professional prostitutes, he also became concerned about the publicity given to what he called the "prostitute prison camp aspect" of the quarantine hospitals. He believed that this characterization worked against the effort to rehabilitate the women and branded all of them as prostitutes. Vonderlehr also recognized that the rehabilitation side of the work was an important justification for the quarantine hospitals, especially as there were "important social and economic reasons why an attempt should be made to salvage this woman power in war time." PHS staff also emphasized that the detention and treatment centers maintained with Lanham Act funds could not be penal institutions, and that any patients incarcerated in them who did not have infectious venereal disease should be removed.[83]

As the war progressed, some of the rapid treatment centers began to admit male patients as well, although the population remained overwhelmingly female throughout the conflict. One 1944 study of 146 patients in a Washington, DC, center, for example, showed that 119 were women and only 27 men. By 1944, Parran noted in an article in *Look Magazine* that men and children were also being admitted to the centers, although the main focus of the article was still on women.[84]

PENICILLIN IN THE TREATMENT OF SYPHILIS

As noted above, penicillin was becoming more widely available for the treatment of syphilis and gonorrhea by the latter part of the war, and the drug was beginning to have a significant impact on the therapy for these diseases. Alexander Fleming had accidentally discovered the antibacterial properties of the *Penicillium* mold in 1928 and realized that a substance produced by the mold (that he called penicillin) might have therapeutic value as a topical agent against disease-causing bacteria. It was not until the early 1940s, however, that researchers at Oxford University in England isolated a relatively pure form of Fleming's penicillin and were able to demonstrate its efficacy as an internal chemotherapeutic agent in animals and then in human clinical trials. The United States government gave high priority to the development of penicillin on a large-scale for use in the war effort, as the drug was proving to be the most potent antibacterial substance known to date. At first supplies were limited and mostly reserved for military use, but by 1944 innovations introduced in American government, university and industry laboratories had greatly increased the yield and available supply of penicillin. In April 1945, all restrictions on its distribution in the United States were removed.[85]

In 1943, investigators at the Mayo Clinic showed that penicillin was effective against gonorrhea bacilli that were resistant to the sulfa drugs, thus giving physicians another weapon against this venereal disease. PHS physician John Mahoney and his colleagues at the Venereal Disease Research Laboratory in the PHS hospital at Staten Island, New York, soon confirmed these results. But Mahoney also decided to divert a small amount of his limited supply of the drug from the gonorrhea research to test it against syphilis. According to a coworker of Mahoney, the drug was first tried against the spirochetes that cause syphilis *in vitro* (i.e., outside of the body in a test tube or other apparatus) and failed to show any activity. Fortunately, the Staten Island investigators proceeded to the next step in trying penicillin *in vivo* (i.e., in the living body) in syphilitic rabbits.[86]

The results of limited animal tests were so encouraging that Mahoney decided to move ahead to clinical experiments. He justified this early move to testing on humans because penicillin appeared to be generally nontoxic and no harm would be done if the drug did not work and he had to return to arsenic therapy. In 1943, it had not yet been recognized that penicillin could produce serious allergic side effects in some patients.[87]

In June 1943, Mahoney and his colleagues began their clinical study with four patients. The results were very promising, and the Staten Island group gave a preliminary report of the work at a national meeting. Although they were cautious in their report of the results, especially since the study had involved only four patients, their paper created great excitement. Microbiologist Gladys Hobby, who heard the presentation of the paper, later recalled:

> I have a mental image of the room where I first heard Mahoney and his associates describe their results on the use of penicillin in the treatment of syphilis. The room was crowded. Loudspeakers and projection equipment were not as sophisticated then as now. Everyone strained to hear what was said, and the impact was electrifying. By then much had been written on penicillin, but no one had expected that an antibacterial agent would be active against spirochetes as well. Hearing John Mahoney describe the effect of penicillin on the course of syphilitic lesions was overwhelming.[88]

The story was picked up by the popular press as well. In an article headed "New Magic Bullet," *Time* discussed how Mahoney, in a "jam-packed session" of the meeting, announced that "penicillin had apparently cured four cases of early syphilis." Dr. Mahoney, according to the story, was "stunned" by the results. The magazine also reported Mahoney's cautious statement that penicillin would have to be tested in a large number of cases over a long period of time before it could be considered a cure for syphilis, but even given the limitations of the study, the results generated high hopes for this new drug against an old disease. One doctor who took to the floor to comment on the paper at the meeting was carried away by his enthusiasm to exult, "This is probably the most significant paper ever presented in the medical field."[89] At another conference a month later, a PHS physician referred to the work of Mahoney and his colleagues as "overshadowing anything that has happened in syphilis control since the days of Ehrlich."[90]

The results of the limited study at Staten Island were promising enough to lead to the organization of a large-scale, national clinical trial of penicillin in the treatment of syphilis. Initially, eight civilian venereal disease clinics, along with one each from the Army, Navy, and Public Health Service, participated in the study, but additional facilities were later included. Not surprisingly, the Staten Island PHS hospital, where Mahoney and his colleagues were located, was one of the original sites for the study. In September 1944, Mahoney and other participants in the study published papers describing their results with over 1400 cases. They were able to demonstrate that penicillin treatment led to the disappearance of the spirochete from open lesions, the healing of those lesions, and a reversal of the blood serologic response from positive to negative (presumably due to the elimination of spirochetes from the blood). Further clinical trials confirmed the place of penicillin as the treatment of choice for syphilis.[91]

On June 26, 1944, the U.S. Army adopted penicillin as the routine treatment for syphilis. Penicillin allowed military physicians to get men suffering from venereal disease back to being available for combat quickly. The infected men remained ambulatory and began to convalesce almost immediately after treatment was begun, so they could be kept close to the front lines and returned to combat as soon as the therapy was completed. At first, however, there was not enough penicillin available to treat all cases that might potentially benefit from it. Penicillin of course had therapeutic value of the treatment of war wounds and various infections diseases other than syphilis and gonorrhea.[92] Physician-ethicist Henry Beecher called attention in a 1969 paper to the problem that military surgeons faced in this situation:

> Allocation of penicillin within the Military was not without its troubles: When the first sizable shipment arrived at the North African Theatre of Operations, U.S.A., in 1943, a decision had to be made between using it for 'sulfa-fast' [sulfa-resistant] gonorrhea or for infected war wounds [its effectiveness against syphilis had not been fully established at the time]. Colonel Edward D. Churchill, Chief Surgical Consultant for that Theatre, made the decision to use the available penicillin for those "wounded" in brothels. Before indignation takes over, one must recall the military manpower shortage of those days. In a week or less, those overcrowding the military hospitals with venereal disease could be restored to health and returned to the battle line.[93]

A moral issue of a different sort was raised by those concerned about the impact of penicillin on sexual mores. As it became more and more obvious that syphilis and gonorrhea could be cured relatively quickly and painlessly with penicillin, some feared that this situation would encourage sexual promiscuity and immorality. One historian has cited a theologian of the period who worried that venereal disease would come to be regarded as strictly a medical problem, with its sociological and moral implications ignored. A graduate student in social work, who completed a research project at a rapid treatment center in 1947, admitted in her dissertation that she could not answer the question of "whether penicillin will be a help or a hindrance to the control of venereal disease; whether by making the treatment so short and effective patients will lose the fear of contracting the disease and will show more laxness in their sexual behavior." A number of public health officials suggested that the quicker and less arduous penicillin treatment could actually lead to an increase in venereal disease. Johns Hopkins bacteriologist Thomas B. Turner, for example, gave a talk at the 1948 ASHA meeting entitled "Penicillin: Help or Hindrance?" in which he not only discussed the successes of the drug against venereal disease, but also cited the loss of fear as a deterrent to exposure. Similar concerns about the undermining of standards of morality had been voiced when Ehrlich's Salvarsan had been introduced to treat syphilis in the early twentieth century.[94]

Concerns about the impact that penicillin might have on sexual behavior did not materially slow the adoption of the drug for the treatment of syphilis and gonorrhea. Nor, however, did the advent of this more effective drug therapy eliminate these diseases or the social and moral issues surrounding them. The final chapter will deal with the history of syphilis since the end of World War II.

SIX

"MAGIC IN THE FORM OF PENICILLIN": SYPHILIS IN AMERICA SINCE WORLD WAR II

THE FALL AND RISE OF SYPHILIS IN POSTWAR AMERICA

As World War II ended, there was new hope that syphilis might finally be controlled with the aid of the "miracle drug" penicillin. Some were even optimistic that the disease might be eradicated. Even before the end of hostilities, a headline in the *New York Times* on May 26, 1944 exclaimed, "End of Syphilis Seen by Use of Penicillin." Among the gains listed in the venereal disease balance sheet published in *Time* in 1946 was that doctors believed that they now had a tool that, with the cooperation of the public, "can almost eradicate venereal disease." In the same optimistic vein, the Deputy Surgeon General of the PHS was reported by the *Chicago Tribune* in early 1946 to have forecast a "swift and final conquest of venereal disease by dosing every man, woman and child in the United States with penicillin," something that he believed would be practical within a few years.[1]

Most public health and social welfare workers were more cautious about predicting the demise of syphilis. In spite of the apparent success of penicillin against the disease, medical officials warned that the drug had not been around long enough to be certain that patients treated with it for syphilis would not suffer relapses. R. A. Vonderlehr and J. R. Heller of the PHS, in their 1946 book on *The Control of Venereal Disease*, reiterated the 1943 caution by syphilis expert John Stokes that it would take a decade or more to know with certainty what penicillin does in syphilis. Theodore Rosenthal, director of New York City's Bureau of Social Hygiene, warned in 1946 at a public health meeting that no final analysis of the place of penicillin in syphilis therapy was yet possible. The following year, Evan Thomas, director of the Bellevue Hospital Rapid Treatment Center, emphasized that it was not yet known whether or not penicillin treatment completely eliminated the syphilis infection. He recommended that patients be reexamined at frequent intervals for at least two years after therapy to detect any relapses.[2]

One author published a pamphlet in 1947 entitled *The Latest So-Called Miracle Cure for Syphilis. Will Penicillin go the Way of Other Cures?* In the publication he talked about the over-optimism that often accompanied new advances in medicine. Even the PHS, he noted, was "not above being infected with the same false optimism which so easily pervades the public mind." The advent of the sulfa drugs, for example, was hailed as "magic." He then added, "Next came more magic in the form of penicillin." While admitting that penicillin was far superior to past treatments for syphilis, he argued that the drug alone could not eliminate the disease. Venereal disease education, prophylaxis, and cleanliness all had a role to play in combating syphilis.[3]

Aside from worries about the long-term effectiveness of penicillin against syphilis, some public health and social hygiene leaders, as we have seen, were concerned that the ease of treatment with the drug would make patients lose their fear of the disease. Vonderlehr and Heller, for example, warned that "should the public assume that the availability of penicillin offers complete freedom to indulge in licentiousness, it is quite within the realm of possibility that venereal disease rates will increase materially." Walter Clarke, executive director of the ASHA, suggested that the easy cure of venereal disease might encourage taking chances in terms of exposure to venereal disease. Syphilis expert John Stokes lamented that if extramarital sex did not lead to significant illness, only a "few intangibles of the spirit" would remain to guide people into moral paths.[4]

Social hygiene leaders had been concerned about a possible increase in venereal disease after the war even before the conflict ended. In January 1945, for example, Walter Clarke reminded Americans that a decrease in antiprostitution efforts and budgets for venereal disease control following World War I had led to an increase in the incidence of syphilis and gonorrhea. He warned that a similar situation could follow the present conflict if appropriate steps were not taken in advance. Clarke reported that studies made by the ASHA suggested that promoters of commercialized prostitution were waiting to restart their enterprise as soon as the war was over, believing that "then public interest and police and court interference will die down and they will be able to operate at the old stand and in the old way." Social hygiene societies, he urged, had to work for educational campaigns, extension of the May Act, continued repression of prostitution, and adequate funding for venereal disease control programs. Supporters of the ASHA position did succeed after the war ended in having the May Act extended, but they failed in their effort to continue the Social Protection Division, which was terminated in 1946.[5]

In the immediate postwar period, it must have seemed that the situation feared by Clarke had indeed materialized. The Surgeon General of the Navy, for example, complained in 1946 that while the nation had achieved the lowest venereal disease rate in history in 1944, reports were coming in that suggested the rate had apparently doubled in many areas over the past two years. The Army reported that the venereal disease rate among American troops stationed in Europe reached 264 cases per thousand on June 16, 1946, the highest rate since the beginning of the war and probably the highest in American military history up to that time. Weekly reports from Germany in 1946 show that the contraction of venereal disease remained at a high level among American troops for most of that year. Sources from the *Los Angeles Times* to the Chairman of the Senate Subcommittee on Health and Education claimed in 1946 and early 1947 that venereal disease rates had soared since the end of the war. Figures reported by state health departments (excluding known military cases) revealed a rise in cases of primary and secondary syphilis in the United States from about 77,000 in fiscal year 1945 to over 106,000 in fiscal year 1947.[6]

The increase in cases of syphilis and gonorrhea following the war, however, was relatively short-lived. By 1948, the rate of incidence of these two diseases had begun to decline. The battle against syphilis in particular appeared to be turning in favor of medicine. In early 1949, Leonard Scheele, Parran's successor as Surgeon General of the PHS, reported that the number of new cases of the disease had dropped 20 percent over the past two years. He proclaimed that we were no longer fighting a defensive battle against syphilis, but had taken the offensive. Reports from various cities and states showed dropping venereal disease rates at the end of the decade. California reported, for example, that the number of civilian cases of primary and secondary syphilis for June through October of 1950 was 62 percent lower than the number for the corresponding period in 1949. New cases of syphilis in the District of Columbia declined from 1018 in 1948 to 597 in 1949 to 164 in 1950. Cases of infectious syphilis in New York City dropped from 13,401 in 1946 to 5,385 in 1950. The incidence of gonorrhea was on the decline also.[7]

As rates of syphilis and gonorrhea continued to fall until the mid-1950s, it seemed as if these infections were dying diseases and, as Harry Dowling stated, "It was assumed that the war against syphilis was almost over." This optimistic view was in evidence at a meeting in Washington, DC, on May 19, 1953 marking the thirtieth anniversary of the District Social Hygiene Society and the fortieth anniversary of the ASHA. The headline of the story in the next day's *Washington Post* reporting on the meeting proclaimed, "Social Hygienists Say War Against VD is Almost Won." The speakers at the meeting stressed, however, that social hygienists still had a job to do, strengthening family life. One speaker noted that "The social hygienist of the future is he who will improve the social climate of the home and family." Social hygienists had always been at least as interested in moral as in health issues, and so their fight would not end with the defeat of venereal disease. Also in 1953, the Eisenhower administration proposed eliminating the PHS venereal disease program because its job was essentially done. Although supporters of the program managed to save it, its budget was cut almost in half.[8]

At a meeting of the American Academy of Dermatology and Syphilology in Chicago in December 1950, Dr. Paul O'Leary of the Mayo Clinic claimed that syphilis was succumbing so rapidly to modern treatments that the time was not far off when medical students would have to consult textbooks to obtain their only information on the disease. In a book published in 1958, John Mahoney, who had discovered the effectiveness of penicillin against syphilis, argued that the use of antibiotics had dramatically reduced the importance of venereal disease as a public health problem. In discussing the decline in the incidence of syphilis, Mahoney noted that complete eradication of a disease is seldom achieved, "but the present situation may well be the exception."[9]

By the time Mahoney published this statement, however, the tide had already begun to turn. Reports of the death of syphilis, to paraphrase Mark Twain, had been greatly exaggerated. Even in the midst of predictions about the possible eradication of syphilis and other venereal diseases, there were some disturbing signs that the battle was far from over. As early as 1953, some public health officials warned that the volume of undisclosed cases of venereal disease in the country was alarming. James Shafer, who was the chief of the PHS DVD at the time, estimated that there were some two million hidden or inadequately treated cases of syphilis alone. In that same year, cases of syphilis reported in the District of Columbia increased slightly, from 16,239 the previous year to 16,698, although all other venereal diseases continued to decline. By 1956, the signs were more ominous, when statistics from 1955 showed that there had been an increase in the "attack rate" of syphilis or gonorrhea, or both, in twenty-five states and fourteen major cities. Early in 1957, it was reported that there had been a rise in syphilis nationwide in 1956 for the first time since 1948. Although the increase was small, only 4,144 cases out of a total number of over 120,000, the reversal in the downward trend of the disease was a cause for concern to groups such as the ASHA.[10]

While at first slight increases in the venereal disease rate could be viewed as temporary setbacks in the march of medical progress, it soon became apparent that the downward trend in cases of these diseases had indeed been reversed. By 1959, William J. Brown, director of the PHS venereal disease program, proclaimed that the evidence suggested that there had been a steady rise in the nation's venereal disease rate since 1954. He cited especially "shocking" increases among youths fifteen to nineteen years old. In the following year, Brown cited statistics showing an increase in infectious syphilis of 42 percent in the last half of 1959 over the same period in 1958.

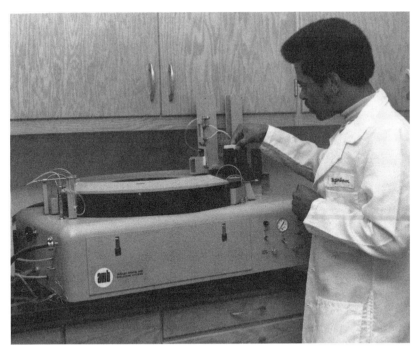

A worker at the Centers for Disease Control and Prevention adjusts an automated fluorescence antibody test machine often used in the identification of the spirochete that causes syphilis [Courtesy of the Centers for Disease Control and Prevention].

The DVD had become a part of the PHS Communicable Disease Center (today known as the Centers for Disease Control and Prevention, or CDC), in Atlanta in 1957, with Brown as its head. Concerned about the rising infection rate, especially among teenagers and young adults, Brown declared war against venereal disease.[11]

As the evidence that venereal disease was on the rise accumulated, public health officials and political leaders became increasingly concerned about the problem, and offered reasons for the increase in the infection rate. With the urgency of the war no longer a factor, and with effective new drugs such as penicillin available, venereal disease control efforts were reduced, a factor cited by many as contributing to the increasing incidence. By July 1953, the last of the rapid treatment centers had been closed. As noted above, the budget of the DVD was cut substantially in the 1950s, hampering efforts to combat these diseases. Federal appropriations for venereal disease control had dropped from $17.37 million in 1949 to $3.0 million in 1955. By 1954, officials of organizations such as the ASHA and the Association of State and Territorial Health Officers were protesting these cuts and warning that they posed a threat to the health of the country's citizens. Historian Allan Brandt has attributed a large part of the blame for the resurgence of venereal disease to this decrease in funding. He pointed out that leading the fight for venereal disease appropriations was not seen by politicians as "a springboard to a wider constituency," and that the "traditional ethic that has emphasized behavioral and moral means as the best way of combating venereal disease, rather than medical and public health approaches," continued to prevail in the United States.[12]

As previously noted, some leaders had expressed concern that the effectiveness of penicillin was creating optimistic views about the impending demise of venereal disease, causing public health officials to relax their control efforts. Others believed that the ease of treatment with penicillin encouraged sexual promiscuity. The increase in venereal disease rates seemed like a confirmation of these fears to many of these individuals. Even DVD chief William Brown was convinced that penicillin was a factor, stating on several occasions that the drug had reduced much of the fear associated with venereal disease. *Time* magazine pointed to a "take-a-chance" attitude with respect to sex among teenagers "now that penicillin has all but eliminated the fear of death and disfigurement." Others, however, such as PHS Deputy Surgeon General William Draper, questioned whether fear of infection had ever been an effective means of preventing the spread of venereal disease. After all, he noted, syphilis and gonorrhea were widespread long before penicillin became available. If one took the argument that penicillin had a negative effect by reducing or eliminating the fear of venereal diseases to its logical conclusion, he asked, did that imply that one should stop treating these diseases, or search for cures that were only partially effective?[13]

Some officials, such as Brown, believed that sexual mores were changing already in the 1950s, especially among teenagers, and argued that values played an important role in the venereal disease story. Brown cited an increase in the number of illegitimate births recorded in the United States, for example, as evidence of increasing social promiscuity. He also pointed to a large number of divorces and broken families as having an impact on teenagers, who might turn to drugs or sex in their "desperate search for love and security." Economic and other factors, he stated, have made the American population more mobile and rootless, and in the experience of the PHS, "some of the most promiscuous persons are transients who spread disease over large areas." The movement of people also "served to water down the established, educational, religious, and family influences." Brown admitted that it is difficult to gauge the effects of changing mores, but he suspected that we might perhaps be living in a time of "relaxed moral responsibility." It appears that even the head of the PHS venereal disease program could not abandon moral considerations and take a purely public health approach to the problem of venereal disease.[14]

With the so-called sexual revolution of the 1960s, more public health officials began to attribute the increasing venereal disease rate, as Allan Brandt has discussed, to what they called the three "p's": permissiveness, promiscuity, and the Pill (i.e., the oral contraceptive). Brandt notes that a fundamental shift in sexual mores did indeed take place in the 1960s, although cautioning that premarital sexual relations had been occurring with increasing frequency over the course of the century. He noted that a greater tolerance of varied sexual practices (e.g., premarital sex, gay sex) developed in the public mind as a new emphasis on individual consent increasingly supplanted "societally imposed moral strictures." By the end of the decade, "an undeniable sexualization of many facets of American life had occurred."[15]

But Brandt rejected the idea espoused by some that a resurgence of venereal disease rates was primarily due to the "sexual revolution" of the 1960s and 1970s. He argued that changes in sexual practices alone could not account for the increase in venereal disease rates. Given the fact that the reversal in the downward trend of venereal disease had begun by about the middle of the 1950s, Brandt would seem to have a point. As noted above, he argued that funding cuts (as well as changes in public health practices in part dictated by these reduced funds) were at least as important in this resurgence, noting that there had been a fairly direct correlation between government spending on venereal disease control and rates of infection.[16]

Brandt also pointed out that in spite of the liberalization of sexual mores in the 1960s, attitudes toward sex education and venereal disease were more resistant to change. Many parents and others opposed the introduction of sex education into the school curriculum. A law was passed in New York in 1969, for example, that removed sex education from the courses eligible for funds under the state's Critical Health Problems Program. Groups such as the Christian Crusade and the John Birch Society fought against sex education in the schools. The Reverend Billy James Hargis, at a rally in Boston in 1969, told the crowd that he did not want "any kid under 12 to hear about lesbians, homosexuals and sexual intercourse." Television shows still refused to deal with subjects such as venereal disease. PHS Surgeon General Luther Terry, in one incident in 1964, tried unsuccessfully to convince the National Broadcasting Company to reinstate cancelled plans for a television drama about a boy who contracts a venereal disease. Even the American Medical Association refused to discuss the use of condoms lest the organization be accused of sanctioning promiscuity. Thomas Parran must have been disappointed to see that there was still a reluctance to candidly discuss syphilis and gonorrhea in postwar America. On one occasion in 1956, six exhibit cases on venereal disease, on display at the Hotel Statler in Washington, DC, were discreetly draped for three hours so as not to upset those attending a Citizens for Eisenhower luncheon meeting, who had to pass the exhibit area to get to their meeting room.[17]

Rather than speculate about complex social and moral issues, physician Ira Schamberg expounded his own medical view of the reduction and subsequent increase in syphilis following World War II. He postulated that in the postwar years, the new "wonder drug" penicillin was widely used for a variety of infections, often even when no specific diagnosis had been made. In this way, many patients with undiagnosed syphilis were incidentally cured of this infection while being treated for other diseases, thus accounting for a decrease in reported cases of the disease. He explained the increasing incidence of the disease that followed from the mid-1950s as due to either the development of resistance against penicillin by the spirochetes that cause syphilis or a decrease in the nonspecific use of penicillin. Others also suggested that the curative or prophylactic action of penicillin given for other purposes played a role in the decrease in venereal disease following the war.[18]

THE CAMPAIGN TO ERADICATE SYPHILIS

Whatever the cause for the resurgence of venereal disease, concern about the problem had reached a point by the beginning of the 1960s that the House Appropriations Committee addressed the issue at its hearings in 1961. The Committee pointed out that syphilis was easy to detect and to cure in its early stages, and so it should be possible to eliminate the disease in the United States. The Committee stated that it would expect the PHS to develop recommendations for a syphilis eradication program by the next year's hearings. As a result of this charge, PHS Surgeon General Luther Terry appointed a Task Force to review the syphilis problem and the existing programs to control the disease, as well as to recommend a course of action to eradicate syphilis as a public health problem. Terry selected D. Leona Baumgartner, Health Commissioner of New York, to chair the group, which held its first meeting on September 13, 1961.[19]

The Task Force delivered its report to the Surgeon General on December 29, 1961. In her letter of transmittal, Baumgartner emphasized that effective action to eliminate syphilis as a public health problem need not await new research advances. She stressed that the basic ingredients to deal with the problem were available, and that health officials dealing with the disease had been "hampered by slim budgets and apathy, both public and professional."[20]

The report called for an intensive and aggressive program based in two general areas of activity, epidemiology and education. In the former area, the Task Force called for an increased effort to find and treat cases of syphilis. This approach would require increased manpower and funding, and would involve such steps as raising the level of syphilis case reporting by private physicians, making available for health department action the results of positive blood tests for syphilis that were currently not being followed up, and intensifying efforts to interview or re-interview syphilis patients for sex contacts. In the education area, the Task Force recommended intensified efforts to educate health professionals and the public, including seminars, conferences, training programs, and energetic use of the mass media. The Task Force believed that if adequate resources were made available, "the epidemic spread of syphilis in this country can be stopped within ten years."[21]

On this basis of this report, President John F. Kennedy in February 1962 called for a 10-year program to eradicate syphilis in this country. This goal was reaffirmed by President Lyndon B. Johnson after he assumed office. In 1965, DVD chief William Brown noted in a speech that to many people the idea of eliminating syphilis in the United States by 1972 seemed like a pipe dream. Yet the nation had also committed itself to landing a man on the moon by 1970, and many who were skeptical about the syphilis eradication goal did not have any doubts about the success of the moon project. Brown told his audience that there were prodigious problems still to be solved in getting a man to the moon and back, whereas in the case of syphilis, we already have reliable means of diagnosing and treating the disease. Although Brown seemed optimistic about the syphilis campaign, he recognized that success depended upon implementing epidemiological and education efforts of the type recommended in the Task Force report.[22]

In 1966, the PHS Public Advisory Committee on Venereal Disease Control (that included all but one of the Task Force members) issued a follow-up to the Task Force report. While praising the efforts that had been made, the group expressed concern that the level of federal funding that was being made available, especially in light of inflation, was not sufficient to fully implement all of the program activities recommended by the Task Force. The Committee also warned that the leveling off and anticipated downward curve of reported syphilis should not be accompanied by a decrease in appropriations for combating the disease before the goal of eradication had been achieved, or that goal would be jeopardized.[23]

The eradication program did at first result in a decreasing rate in the reported cases of infectious syphilis. In its report for fiscal year 1967, for example, the Venereal Disease Program, as the DVD was now called, stated that such cases had declined for the second consecutive year. In fiscal year 1967, the 21,090 cases of primary and secondary syphilis represented a decrease of 6.2 percent from the 22,473 cases of the previous year. Cases of primary and secondary syphilis continued to decline over the next couple of years. But once again those who had predicted the imminent demise of syphilis were proven wrong. In calendar year 1970, cases of primary and secondary syphilis reached 21,982, a jump of almost 3,000 over the previous year. These figures continued to rise through the mid-1970s. In 1972, the target year for eradication of the disease in the United States, there were still 24,429 reported cases of primary and secondary syphilis, a figure higher than the 21,067 cases in calendar year 1962, when the campaign was initiated. The rate had increased slightly from 11.5 to 11.8 per 100,000 population over this period. Clearly the ten-year eradication program had failed.[24]

In the original target year of 1972, a National Commission on Venereal Disease admitted that venereal disease was epidemic in the United States. The Commission called for a massive drive against venereal disease. Their recommendations, however, were strikingly similar to those of the earlier Task Force, involving a combination of increased testing, stricter reporting, better education, and more money.[25]

SYPHILIS IN THE KOREAN AND VIETNAM WARS

As we have seen, venereal disease is a problem that has long plagued military leaders, especially in wartime. The Korean and Vietnam Wars were no exception. Since the focus of this book is on the problem of syphilis as it existed in the United States itself, however, the issue of the disease in American troops serving abroad has not been discussed in detail. In the case of the two major American wars of the second half of the twentieth century, the subject will again be treated briefly, with the reader referred to other sources for more extensive coverage.

In 1948, President Harry Truman appointed a committee composed of educators, clergymen, and civic leaders to study and advise the Department of Defense on matters relating to education, religion, community relations, leisure, and housing in the military. Chaired by Frank Weil, the president of the National Social Welfare Assembly, the group had significant impact through pressuring the military to accept certain social reforms. The Weil Committee argued that the overriding purpose of all information and education in the military should be "to make personnel better citizens, citizens who were impervious to the attack of rival ideologies." In the cold war era, the rival ideology of concern was of course communism.[26]

Closely related to the political indoctrination against communism in the mind of the Weil Committee was the idea that immorality and "godlessness" also undermined democratic ideals. The Committee therefore urged the establishment of wholesome programs to promote character growth and the provision of adequate religious opportunities for service personnel. Therefore, by the late 1940s the military began to emphasize continence and self-discipline over the provision of condoms in its venereal disease program. The typical World War II venereal disease films were replaced by films that advocated a moral approach to the subject. Service personnel who contracted a venereal disease were dealt with more harshly.[27]

Abstract goals, however, were often abandoned when confronted by reality, especially among the troops stationed abroad. By 1950, venereal disease rates were increasing among American troops in Korea. In Pusan, an area where there was a large concentration of troops, it was estimated that there were some eight thousand prostitutes. Dance halls were opened to accommodate the soldiers. In his history of medicine in the Korean War, Albert Cowdrey notes, "After visiting such establishments, soldiers retired with chosen partners to finish the evening in a crib, private home, hotel, or paddy field." Nonpunitive measures were used in the effort to control venereal disease because it was feared that punishment would lead to evasion and self-treatment. The Army set up prophylactic stations to treat the troops. Although the Army held lectures appealing to moral sentiment, they also freely distributed condoms and prophylactic kits to the soldiers. Before and after men went on leave, they were frequently subjected to physical, or "short-arm," inspection. Dr. Hawkeye Pierce, made famous by the popular novel, movie and television show $M^*A^*S^*H$, gave the following instructions for conducting such an inspection:

> You get a chair. You sit on it backwards with your arms clasped behind its back and your chin resting on the top. You gotta have a big cigar in your mouth. You sit there and look. Most of the guys will know what to do. If they don't, you growl, "Skin it and wring it, soldier." Sound mean when you say it. If you think there is a suspicion of venereal disease, you make a gesture with your thumb like Bill Klem [a baseball umpire] calling a guy out at the plate. Then somebody hauls the guy off somewhere.[28]

Venereal disease rates continued to climb in Korea, jumping from 176.8 to 202 cases per thousand troops from September to November of 1952. Korean leaders and the United States Army did not agree on the best tactics for dealing with the problem. The Koreans preferred to informally license brothels and inspect the prostitutes, arguing that the Army's policy of closing down the brothels or placing them off limits merely drove the prostitutes into the streets, where they were harder to control. Military and civil authorities also frequently disagreed on policies toward venereal disease. As noted earlier, the Weil Commission favored dealing with the problem through moral exhortation and providing "wholesome entertainment" for the soldiers, but Army leaders often tended to rely on prophylactic measures.[29]

Even after the end of hostilities in Korea, prostitution and its relationship to venereal disease continued to be an issue with regard to American troops stationed in that country, as discussed in detail by Katharine Moon in her book, *Sex among Allies: Military Prostitution in U.S.–Korea Relations.*[30] Sue Son Yom recorded that "many observers remarked that the Korean was the most 'venereal war' in history." The venereal disease rate in the American military was three times as high in the Korean War as it was in World War II. But that rate was to increase even further in the Vietnam War, to more than double the rate of the Korean War. As Yom claimed, by the time of the Vietnam War, "sexual adventure with foreign women had become an integral part of the modern overseas military experience." Although the official policy of the Department of Defense was to suppress prostitution whenever possible, military leaders realized that it would not be possible to completely eliminate prostitution. This was especially true in situations, as in these two conflicts, where poverty and hardship often forced women into prostitution, or where they could be sold into sexual slavery. Prostitution also flourished in Thailand, the Philippines, Japan (especially Okinawa), and Hong Kong, which were visited by American soldiers on leave from Vietnam.[31]

In Vietnam, as in Korea, American military leaders also recognized that moral persuasion was not enough to control the sexual behavior of the troops, and they tolerated and even became involved in the business of prostitution. Military brothels had been established in Vietnam by the French. By the time that the Americans replaced the French, conditions in South Vietnam had deteriorated to the point where prostitution became the only viable means of earning a living for thousands of South Vietnamese women. Eventually the American military, like the French military before it, actually became involved in supplying women to the troops. As Susan Brownmiller explained:

> The American military got into the prostitution business by degrees, an escalation process linked to the escalation of the war. Underlying the escalation was the assumption that men at war required the sexual use of women's bodies... Military brothels on Army base camps ("Disneylands" or "boom-boom parlors") were built by decision of a division commander, a two-star general, and were under the direct operational control of a brigade commander with the rank of colonel. Clearly, Army brothels in Vietnam existed by the grace of Army Chief of Staff William C. Westmoreland, the United States Embassy in Saigon, and the Pentagon.[32]

One Army officer used the brothel of his unit not only to control venereal disease, but also to promote camaraderie and relieve racial tensions in the unit. Officers, however, were not expected to utilize prostitution services. These services were intended for the enlisted men, to keep them happy. Unlike the Army, the Marine Corps apparently attempted to enforce a relatively strict moral code.[33]

In spite of efforts to control venereal disease, including the establishment of the "official" brothels, the venereal disease rate remained high. In response to this increasing rate of disease, the educational film *Where the Girls Are—VD in Southeast Asia* was released in early 1969. The film was produced for the Air Force, but was later adopted for use by the Army as well. It was the only major feature produced by the military about this topic during the Vietnam War. *Where the Girls Are* did not attempt to moralize about sex. In fact, it basically assumed that soldiers would inevitably engage in sexual acts. Rather, the film was designed to make the men knowledgeable about venereal disease and its clinical management and control. The film, in the words of Yom, "embodied the contradictions of U.S. military policy, which on the one hand recommended the formal elimination of prostitution yet on the other acceded to its practical demands."[34]

Since a high venereal disease rate was counted against the merit rating of a battalion, commanders went to ingenious lengths to try to lower their counts. In spite of this practice, the reported rate was still exceptionally high. The venereal disease rate in the Army reached 325 per thousand troops per year. Gonorrhea was much more common than syphilis in the military during the Vietnam War. At Camp Lejune in North Carolina, a Marine Corps base, there were 67 cases of syphilis and 376 cases of gonorrhea in 1965. Physicians at a United States Air Force hospital in Vietnam reported that they rarely saw cases of syphilis. They speculated that the relative rarity of syphilis was due to the high doses of penicillin used to treat gonorrhea, which was common among the patients.[35]

One widespread legend among American servicemen in Vietnam was that of an incurable form of venereal disease, sometimes referred to as the "black syph" or the "black rose," among other names. Rumors circulated among the troops that men who contracted this dreaded, untreatable disease were reported as dead and sent to secluded islands to live out their days because it was feared that returning them to the United States could lead to an epidemic. One version of this myth held that this strain of the disease had come about because the frequent and continued use of penicillin among prostitutes in Vietnam had led to the creation of a condition that was resistant to treatment with antibiotics. Some individuals suggested that the military might have actually invented and promoted such stories to discourage servicemen from having sex with prostitutes. Whatever the origin of the "black syph" legend, like most rumors the story probably became more extreme as it was retold many times.[36]

SYPHILIS IN THE ERA OF AIDS

The failure of the 1960s campaign to eradicate syphilis did at least generate a renewed push to do a better job of controlling venereal disease. In 1972, the original target year for syphilis eradication, a CDC official believed that "the promised land" of venereal disease control was just ahead (a prediction that had been made before). He proclaimed that it was time to stop complaining about lack of funds, shortage of people, etc. and get the job done. The funds devoted to the program were increased somewhat, and a commitment was made to implement a national program of tracing contacts. The CDC also launched a campaign against gonorrhea, which seemed to be raging uncontrolled and which previously had not received the attention that syphilis had. Ironically, this renewed venereal disease effort was happening at the same time that the previously discussed Tuskegee Syphilis Study was coming to light in the public press.[37]

Presumably the CDC's renewed efforts played a part in the reversal of the increasing venereal disease rate that soon took place. In 1973–1974, the number of reported cases of primary and secondary syphilis decreased for the first time in six years, dropping 1.4 percent from 1972–1973. Although gonorrhea cases increased by 8 percent over this period, this figure was lower than the increases of the previous two years. The downward trend continued, as the number of cases of primary and secondary syphilis declined by about 1,800 from 1975 to 1976, and cases of gonorrhea increased by only one-half of one percent over that same period. By the end of the decade, however, the number of cases of primary and secondary syphilis was beginning to creep up again, and the number of gonorrhea cases was still holding steady.[38]

As the 1980s dawned, however, the nation's attention was riveted by a new and deadly sexually transmitted disease, Acquired Immunodeficiency Syndrome (AIDS). First recognized in 1981, the disease was soon shown to be transmitted by a virus, the Human Immunodeficiency Virus (HIV). Although other sexually transmitted diseases, such as herpes and chlamydia, had come to be recognized in the preceding decades, none posed the threat that AIDS did. At first there was no treatment for the disease, which was invariably fatal. Syphilis and gonorrhea, by comparison, did not seem so bad. Nevertheless, they continued to represent significant public health problems.[39]

Because the AIDS epidemic first surfaced in the gay community, many people originally saw it as a disease associated with the homosexual lifestyle, and especially with unprotected sex with multiple partners. It was soon shown, however, that heterosexuals could also contract and transmit the disease, and that it could be transmitted through blood transfusions or the sharing of needles among drug users as well as by sexual acts.

Relatively little attention had been paid to the matter of sexually transmitted diseases such as syphilis among gays before the 1960s. The fact that homosexual acts could cause syphilis or gonorrhea was occasionally mentioned in the medical literature at least as early as the eighteenth century in Europe, although William Benemann found only one veiled mention of homosexuality in his examination of twenty-nine medical books published in the United States between 1787 and 1820.[40] The subject continued to receive little attention in the American medical literature before the mid-twentieth century.[41] As concerns developed about the increasing rate of venereal disease in the late 1950s and early 1960s, however, gays began to receive increased attention from the medical community. Public health workers began to notice an increase in the percentage of males among those infected with syphilis. In Los Angeles, for example, prior to 1956 under 70 percent of the primary and secondary syphilis cases were males. By 1960, that figure had risen to 91.4 percent. The increase was especially marked among white males, where the numbers increased from 34 to 386 over this time period, a jump of over 1000 percent.

The evidence seemed to suggest that gay men accounted for a significant part of this increase in the male population. For example, of the 419 males treated for syphilis by private physicians and clinics in Los Angeles in 1960 who revealed the identities of their sexual partners, 77.3 percent named only male contacts and another 4.3 percent named both male and female contacts. The New York Medical College reported that 43 percent of males treated in its clinics for primary and secondary syphilis at that time were homosexuals. In addition, by 1963 thirty-three states and sixty-four cities stated that homosexuality was contributing to an increasing percentage of venereal disease cases (although it is not clear on what evidence these conclusions were based). Whether syphilis was actually increasing among gay men, or whether gay men were simply more willing to reveal their sexual preferences by the 1960s, it is clear that public health officials began to pay more attention to the spread of the disease in the gay community. Although officials admitted that they had much less information about lesbians, they generally believed that little venereal disease was transmitted by this group.[42]

Given the fact that homosexual acts were prohibited by law in many states, public health leaders realized that gays diagnosed with syphilis might be reluctant to reveal their contacts. In the military, the admission of a homosexual act could lead to a court martial and severe punishment, and doctor-patient confidentiality was not maintained. Some public health workers emphasized the importance of maintaining a nonjudgmental, sympathetic, and understanding attitude in interviewing gay venereal disease patients. Another issue cited by health officials was the belief of some homosexuals that syphilis could not be transmitted by anal or oral sex.[43]

Hopes for eradicating syphilis continued to be frustrated. As noted above, the disease was on the increase again as the 1980s opened, although this problem was soon overshadowed by the advent of AIDS. The pendulum began to swing the other way again in the 1990s. The rate of primary and secondary syphilis in the United States declined by 89 percent from 1990 to 2000, reaching the lowest rate since reporting began in 1941. This low rate, along with the fact that the majority of cases were concentrated in a relatively small number of geographic areas (the South and certain urban centers), once again raised hopes that the disease could be eradicated. In October 1999, PHS Surgeon General David Satcher announced the launch of a new National Plan to Eliminate Syphilis from the United States.[44]

The 1999 plan emphasized that over 50 percent of cases of infectious (primary and secondary) syphilis were concentrated in just twenty-eight counties in the United States, the majority of them in the South. The disease also disproportionately affected African Americans living in poverty, in spite of the fact that the black: white ratio for syphilis had decreased by almost one-half since the early 1990s. Other groups identified as being disproportionately affected by the disease included drug users, people exchanging sex for money or drugs, men who have sex with men, and minority and migrant populations affected by racism, high unemployment rates, poor educational opportunities, and poverty. The plan involved five strategies for eliminating syphilis, three of which were basically time-tested public health methods that had also been a part of the 1960s syphilis eradication campaign: enhanced surveillance, expanded clinical and laboratory services, and enhanced health promotion. The published plan claimed, however, that the other two approaches—strengthened community involvement and partnerships and rapid outbreak response—would be new in many parts of the country.[45]

Once again, however, syphilis proved to be remarkably resilient. Cases of primary and secondary syphilis in the United States rose by 2 percent in 2000 and 2001, reversing the downward trend in effect during the previous decade. Rates among African Americans and women of all races declined, but there were increases in this period in other groups, such as gay and bisexual men. By 2004, there were 7,980 reported cases of primary and secondary syphilis, an increase of some 2,000 cases over the number in 2000. While these numbers were still low by historical standards (e.g., there were over 50,000 cases in 1990), they illustrated the difficulty of completely eliminating the disease.[46]

By the time that the 1999 plan was issued, public health officials were already aware that the rise and fall of syphilis appeared to be cyclic. The plan stressed that there was only a short window of opportunity available to try to eliminate the disease while cases were still declining. As we have seen, that effort did not succeed, as cases began to climb again in the first decade of the twenty-first century. In 2005, scientists at Imperial College in Britain published a study providing evidence that the cycle of syphilis infection that peaks at eight- to eleven-year intervals is a natural cycle that is independent of sexual behaviors. The authors examined syphilis data from sixty-eight American cities over a fifty-year period to clearly show the cyclic nature of the disease. By contrast, gonorrhea, which is also sexually transmitted, did not show a similar cyclical pattern. Gonorrhea rates steadily rose from the 1950s to the 1970s, and then steadily declined. The British investigators predicted that syphilis incidence would continue to rise in the United States for the next few years because of the natural cycle of the disease.

The Imperial College scientists also were able to offer a plausible explanation for their findings. The difference between syphilis and gonorrhea could be explained on the basis of immunity. People who recover from syphilis retain some immunity against the disease for a period of time, whereas this is not the case with gonorrhea. When syphilis rates are high, the disease produces a population with a relatively high degree of immunity, and infection rates fall. But as the population evolves, the number of susceptible individuals increases, and so does the infection rate. The British investigators used a computer model to show that the time from one peak to another should be about a decade, as observed. Thus, instead of the peak in syphilis rates in the early 1970s being due to the sexual revolution, or that of the 1980s to the spread of crack cocaine, as some have postulated, it may be that these peaks were just part of the natural cycle of the disease. The Imperial College group did not claim that sexual behavior had no influence on the number of people infected, but concluded that the regular ups and downs were an intrinsic property of the disease itself.[47]

Success in eradicating a disease, such as eliminating smallpox worldwide and polio in many countries, has largely been based on the availability of a vaccine against the disease. However, no vaccine exists against syphilis. As we have seen, there were efforts to develop such a vaccine as early as the nineteenth century, but without success. The search for a suitable vaccine has continued up to the present day. Like smallpox, syphilis has no animal reservoir, i.e., humans are the only natural host (even though the disease has been artificially induced in some animals). Therefore, eliminating the disease from humans should result in its eradication. However, technical difficulties, such as the fact that the spirochete could not be propagated *in vitro* (i.e., outside the body) and the organism's unusual cellular architecture, hindered the development of a successful vaccine.[48] Although the spirochete does stimulate the body to produce antibodies that protect the victim against further infection, this immunity is short-lived. Scientists have studied the immunological reaction to syphilis in an effort to better understand it and utilize this knowledge in the production of a vaccine. At various times, success has appeared to be within sight. In the 1950s, for example, experiments on volunteers at Sing Sing prison in Ossining, New York, involving injections with dead spirochetes at first seemed promising, but eventually were unsuccessful. In the late 1960s, medical researchers at the University of California Los Angeles (UCLA) used gamma rays to "stun" spirochetes. Since earlier attempts to produce a syphilis vaccine with spirochetes killed by heat or chemicals had failed, the UCLA investigators hoped that they might succeed with a vaccine involving a microorganism weakened enough by radiation so that it would not induce the disease but still active enough to produce immunity. In 1973, James Miller at UCLA did have some success with this procedure when he inoculated rabbits with spirochetes killed by gamma radiation and showed that this vaccine provided protection against syphilis for at least a year. However, achieving this level of immunity required sixty intravenous injections over thirty-seven weeks, a procedure that was too long and invasive to be practical in humans. Various other methods were tried in the following years that sometimes initially seemed promising, but ultimately failed. Even the successful growth of the spirochete *in vitro* for the first time in 1976 did not lead to a vaccine.[49]

Hopes for a syphilis vaccine were once again raised in the late 1990s when the genome of the spirochete was decoded. Scientists believed that knowledge of the complete DNA sequence of the microorganism might provide them with the clues that they needed to produce an effective vaccine. The DNA of the genome codes for the synthesis of proteins in the organism. Researchers recognized that proteins on the surface of the spirochete were probably targeted by the immune cells of the body for attack. If they could identify these proteins and separate them from the microorganism, they might be able to stimulate a concentrated immune system reaction against these compounds, without having to introduce the spirochete itself into the body. In 2000, Sheila Lukehart and her colleagues at the University of Washington searched the spirochete genome to identify such proteins. Three of the proteins identified and isolated showed promising results.[50]

Unfortunately, immunization produced by the use of such proteins has thus far induced only partial protection against syphilis. As of the writing of this book, there is still no effective vaccine against syphilis. The search continues for molecules on the outer membrane surface of the spirochete that would lead to the production of a successful vaccine.[51]

The AIDS epidemic has heightened concerns about syphilis because of the interaction between the two diseases. Various studies strongly suggest that syphilis, because of ulcers produced on the genitals, promotes the transmission of HIV infection. It is also possible that syphilis is a cofactor in the progression of HIV infection to the disease AIDS. Coinfection with syphilis and HIV is not uncommon. Because of a weakened immune system in patients infected with HIV, syphilis may progress more rapidly and the risk of relapse may be higher in these individuals. There are even a handful of researchers, distinctly in the minority, who have suggested that the spirochete of syphilis is the real cause of AIDS.[52]

With reported cases of primary and secondary syphilis on the increase in the middle of the first decade of the twenty-first century, the CDC issued a revision of its 1999 plan to eradicate syphilis in May 2006. The campaign was by then being referred to as the Syphilis Elimination Effort (SEE). Based on a report compiled by CDC consultants in 2005, the revised plan did not radically change the basic strategies of the original document, but made some modifications in programmatic implementation based on changing circumstances and lessons learned. For example, the recent resurgence of syphilis among men who have sex with men suggested that more attention be devoted to this group. The new plan also called for other changes, such as adopting a more holistic approach that took into consideration the social determinants of disease transmission and making use of the Internet. The plan set interim targets for 2010 for the reduction of rates of primary and secondary syphilis, among other goals, and emphasized that it "should not be seen as a rigid blueprint for eliminating syphilis instantly." It remains to be seen whether this latest effort to eradicate syphilis in the United States will succeed where earlier campaigns have failed.[53]

In the 1980s, as the country and the world were still adjusting to the reality of the AIDS epidemic and how to deal with it, historian Allan Brandt called attention in several publications to similarities between AIDS and previous sexually transmitted diseases, especially syphilis. These analogues include "the pervasive fear of contagion; concerns about casual transmission; the stigmatization of victims; the conflicts between protecting public health and assuring civil liberties; the search for magic bullets." Although clearly recognizing that AIDS was not syphilis, and that one could not predict its future based on the history of syphilis and other venereal diseases, Brandt did argue that there were "lessons" that could be learned from the past.[54]

More recently (2001), Perry Treadwell also compared syphilis and AIDS and the reaction to these diseases. Treadwell sounded less sanguine about gleaning lessons from the past, noting that the human response to the AIDS epidemic "proves that society has learned little about coping with sexually transmitted diseases." Among the similarities between the histories of syphilis and AIDS pointed out by Treadwell are the fact that some people believed when the diseases first appeared that they were a judgment from God, the tendency to blame a particular group for the malady,

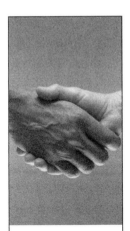

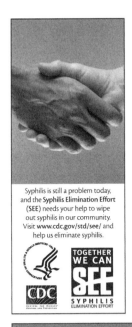

Syphilis is still a problem today, and the **Syphilis Elimination Effort** (SEE) needs your help to wipe out syphilis in our community. Visit **www.cdc.gov/std/see/** and help us eliminate syphilis.

Syphilis is still a problem today, and it is in our community. The **Syphilis Elimination Effort** (SEE) is a national initiative to eliminate syphilis and wipe out one of our nation's biggest racial disparities in health. If you are a health care provider, a community leader, or a policy maker, find out what you can do to eliminate syphilis in our community. Visit **www.cdc.gov/std/see/** and help us eliminate syphilis.

The **Syphilis Elimination Effort** (SEE) is a national initiative to eliminate syphilis and wipe out one of our nation's biggest racial disparities in health. If you are a health care provider, a community leader, or a policy maker, your participation is greatly needed. Visit **www.cdc.gov/std/see/** and help us eliminate syphilis now.

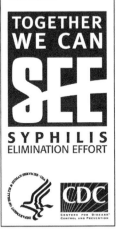

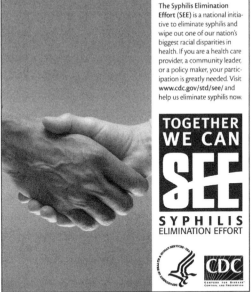

Advertisements for the Centers for Disease Control and Prevention's current campaign to eliminate syphilis [Courtesy of the Centers for Disease Control and Prevention].

fearfulness of the disease, the initial speed of infection, calls for quarantining the infected, fear that a treatment or vaccination would encourage promiscuity, and opposition to sex education.[55]

Certainly the story of syphilis as discussed here shows troubling similarities to the initial reaction to AIDS, such as the reluctance of many to talk openly about the disease and its sexual aspects and a tendency on the part of some to blame victims for bringing the disease upon themselves by "immoral" behavior." There also seemed to be a need to find scapegoats. The French blamed the Italians for syphilis and vice versa. Many Europeans eventually came to blame Indians from the Americas for the disease. Women, especially prostitutes and those who were considered promiscuous, bore the brunt of the blame for the spread of venereal disease. In the case of AIDS, the initial focus was on homosexuals, as AIDS was considered a "gay disease." Later other groups, such as Haitians and intravenous drug users, were also singled out as transmitters of the infection.

Opposition on the part of segments of the population to sex education, including a hesitancy to talk candidly about sexually transmitted diseases and how to avoid them, also marks the history of both syphilis and AIDS. The problems faced by PHS Surgeon General C. Everett Koop and other public health officials in dealing with AIDS in the 1980s, for example, remind one of this issues faced by Koop's predecessor, Thomas Parran, with respect to syphilis. Like Parran before him, Koop was criticized for openly talking about a sexually transmitted disease. Koop was especially attacked for promoting prophylaxis, and was dubbed the "Condom King" by some. His 1986 report on AIDS and the AIDS brochure that he sent to every American household in the following year were controversial because of their candid discussion of the issues surrounding the disease.[56]

Striking a balance between civil liberties and public health is also a theme that figures in the history of both syphilis and AIDS, though it is not one that is limited to sexually transmitted diseases. The rights of certain individuals have been curtailed for centuries in the name of public health, as for example in quarantining ships or neighborhoods where there has been an infectious disease outbreak. The Irish-American cook Mary Mallon ("Typhoid Mary") was forcibly confined for a significant portion of her life because she was a typhoid carrier. We have seen that historically prostitutes with venereal disease were sometimes quarantined and subjected to forced treatment in various countries. In the United States during World Wars I and II, thousands of women with a venereal disease (or suspected of having one) were detained in quarantine hospitals because they were perceived as a threat to the health of soldiers and essential war workers. Although no large-scale quarantine of those infected with HIV occurred in the United States, such measures were discussed. A *Los Angeles* Times poll in 1985 revealed that a slight majority of Americans favored the quarantine of AIDS patients. Other civil liberties issues were also raised with respect to AIDS, as in the controversy over whether or not to close gay bathhouses. Another measure considered by the Reagan Administration, although never implemented, was mandatory testing for AIDS. In the case of both AIDS and syphilis, individuals were also understandably concerned about the confidentiality of test results.[57]

Brandt has identified four lessons that we can learn from the history of sexually transmitted diseases, all of which have some relevance to our understanding of the AIDS epidemic. These lessons are: (1) fear of disease will powerfully influence medical approaches and public health policy; (2) education will not control the AIDS epidemic; (3) compulsory public health measures will not control the epidemic; and (4) the development of effective treatments and vaccines will not immediately or easily end the AIDS epidemic. He goes on to give examples to justify these conclusions. The discussion of the history of syphilis in this book supports many of Brandt's points. For example, involuntary quarantine of prostitutes and "promiscuous" women in World War I and World War II did not control the venereal disease problem, nor did mandatory premarital testing for syphilis. The introduction of penicillin, with its ability to cure syphilis and gonorrhea quickly and painlessly, did not lead to the eradication of these diseases, in spite of high expectations that it would. Brandt made clear that he was not implying that nothing would work, but suggesting that no single avenue would be likely to lead to success and that there are no simple answers. Each intervention (whether involving education, testing, research, etc.) requires sophisticated research to understand its potential impact, and needs to be evaluated in terms of its effectiveness as a measure to control the disease.[58]

Hopefully an understanding of the history of syphilis can inform our public health approaches not only to AIDS, but to other infectious diseases as well. There was a period during the 1960s when medical leaders believed that we had almost conquered infectious diseases, and could devote our attention more fully to chronic diseases such as cancer and heart disease. This view proved to be overly optimistic. First of all, pathogenic microorganisms proved to be much more resilient to our "magic bullets" that we initially realized, as strains resistant to our drugs evolved. The public is well aware by now, for example, of the health problems involving drug-resistant tuberculosis and methicillin-resistant *Staphylococcus aurea* (MRSA). New infectious diseases, in addition to AIDS, have come onto the scene in recent decades, including Ebola fever, severe acute respiratory syndrome (SARS), and West Nile virus. Scientists speak of emerging and reemerging infectious diseases. Even some infectious diseases that have been known to mankind for ages and for which preventive measures and treatments exist, such as malaria and cholera, still take a high toll of lives in many areas of the world.[59]

We cannot predict the future from the past. The history of syphilis will not give us an exact blueprint for dealing with other infectious diseases that confront us today. History can help us to understand, however, how disease (and our reaction to it) is shaped by its social, cultural, and historical context. As Brandt has noted, "It is an understanding of this process which gives the historical record relevance and meaning."[60] It is my hope that the reader of this book will not only have been enlightened about the history of syphilis, but will also have acquired a broader appreciation of disease as a social as well as a medical construct and of the way in which social and cultural factors influence our understanding of and reaction to any given disease.

NOTES

INTRODUCTION

1. Thomas Parran and R. A. Vonderlehr, *Plain Words about Venereal Disease* (New York: Reynal and Hitchcock, 1941), p. 4.

2. Theodor Rosebury, *Microbes and Morals: The Strange Story of Venereal Disease* (New York: Viking Press, 1971), p. xvi.

3. James T. Patterson, "How Do We Write the History of Disease," *Health and History* 1 (1998): 8–28; Charles E. Rosenberg and Janet Golden, eds., *Framing Disease: Studies in Cultural History* (New Brunswick, NJ: Rutgers University Press, 1992).

4. Naomi Rogers, *Dirt and Disease: Polio before FDR* (New Brunswick, NJ: Rutgers University Press, 1992), pp. 1–8 (quotation on p. 7); Naomi Rogers, "Dirt, Flies, and Immigrants: Explaining the Epidemiology of Poliomyelitis, 1900–1916," *Journal of the History of Medicine* 44 (1989): 486–505.

5. Barbara Bates, *Bargaining for Life: A Social History of Tuberculosis, 1876–1938* (Philadelphia. PA: University of Pennsylvania Press, 1992), p. 3; David McBride, *From TB to AIDS: Epidemics among Urban Blacks since 1900* (Albany, NY: State University of New York Press, 1991), pp. 1–6.

6. Tristram Engelhardt, Jr., "The Disease of Masturbation: Values and the Concept of Disease," *Bulletin of the History of Medicine* 48 (1974): 234–248; Bert Hansen, "American Physicians' 'Discovery' of Homosexuals, 1880–1900: A New Diagnosis in a Changing Society," in Rosenberg and Golden, *Framing Disease*, pp. 104–133.

7. Tony Gould, *A Disease Apart: Leprosy in the Modern World* (New York: St. Martin's Press, 2005); Zachary Gussow, *Leprosy, Racism, and Public Health: Social Policy in Chronic Disease*

Control (Boulder, CO: Westview Press, 1989); John Parascandola, "'An Exile in My Own Country': The Confinement of Leprosy Patients at the United States National Leprosarium," *Medicina nei Secoli* 10 (1998): 111–125; Luke Demaitre, *Leprosy in Premodern Medicine: A Malady of the Whole Body* (Baltimore, MD: Johns Hopkins University Press, 2007); Michelle T. Moran, *Colonizing Leprosy: Imperialism and the Politics of Public Health in the United States* (Chapel Hill, NC: University of North Carolina Press, 2007).

    8. Celia W. Dugger, "South Africa Confines the Ill to Fight Severe TB," *New York Times* March 25, 2008, pp. A1 and A10.

CHAPTER ONE

    1. Quoted in Claude Quétel, *History of Syphilis*, translated into English by Judith Braddock and Brian Pike (Baltimore, MD: Johns Hopkins University Press, 1990), p. 42.

    2. On the early Italian Wars, see David Nicolle, *Fornovo 1495: France's Bloody Fighting Retreat* (Westport, CT: Praeger, 2005); F. L. Taylor, *The Art of War in Italy 1494–1529* (London: Greenhill, 1993).

    3. Quétel, *History of Syphilis*, pp. 10–15; Jon Arrizabalaga, John Henderson, and Roger French, *The Great Pox: The French Disease in Renaissance Europe* (New Haven, CT: Yale University Press, 1997), pp. 25–27.

    4. Quétel, *History of Syphilis*, pp. 10–12; Roze Hentschell, "Luxury and Lechery: Hunting the French Pox in Early Modern England," in *Sins of the Flesh: Responding to Sexual Disease in Early Modern Europe*, ed. Kevin Siena (Toronto: Centre for Reformation and Renaissance Studies, 2005), pp. 133–157.

    5. On syphilis and its relation to the "Great Pox," see Arrizabalaga et al., *The Great Pox*, pp. 1–19.

    6. Darin Hayton, "Joseph Grünpeck's Astrological Explanation of the French Disease," in Siena, *Sins of the Flesh*, pp. 81–106; Theodor Rosebury, *Microbes and Morals: The Strange Story of Venereal Disease* (New York: Viking Press, 1971), p. 24.

    7. Arrizabalaga et al., *The Great Pox*, p. 50.

    8. Quétel, *History of Syphilis*, p. 33.

    9. Arrizabalaga et al., *The Great Pox*, pp. 6, 14, 24.

    10. Ibid., pp. 107–112; Hayton, "Grünpeck's Astrological Explanation."

    11. Quétel, *History of Syphilis*, pp. 34–35; Sheldon Watts, *Epidemics and History: Disease, Power and Imperialism* (New Haven, CT: Yale University Press, 1997), p. 130.

    12. Quoted in Quétel, *History of Syphilis*, p. 35.

    13. Ibid., pp. 35–36.

    14. Diane Cady, "Linguistic Dis-ease: Foreign Language as Sexual Disease in Early Modern England," in Siena, *Sins of the Flesh*, pp. 159–186; Anna Foa, "The New and the Old: The Spread of Syphilis (1494–1530)," translated into English by Carole C. Gallucci, in *Sex and Gender in Historical Perspective*, eds. Edward Muir and Guido Ruggiero (Baltimore, MD: Johns Hopkins University Press, 1990), pp. 26–45.

    15. Arrizabalaga et al., *The Great Pox*, p. 12.

    16. Quétel, *History of Syphilis*, p. 37.

    17. C. Meyer, C. Jung, T. Kohl, A. Poenicke, A. Poppe, and K. W. Alt, "Syphilis 2001—A Paleontological Reappraisal," *Homo* 53 (2002): 39–58 (quotation on p. 39).

18. Mary Lucas Powell and Della Collins Cook, eds., *The Myth of Syphilis: The Natural History of Treponematosis in North America* (Gainesville, FL: University Press of Florida, 2005).

19. Della Collins Cook and Mary Lucas Powell, "Piecing the Puzzle Together: North American Treponematosis in Overview," in Powell and Cook, *The Myth of Syphilis*, pp. 442–479 (quotation on p. 477).

20. John Noble Wilford, "Genetic Study Bolsters Columbus Link to Syphilis," *New York Times*, January 15, 2008, p. D2.

21. Meyer et al.,"Syphilis 2001."

22. Quétel, *History of Syphilis*, pp. 22–23; Arrizibalaga et al., *The Great Pox*, pp. 129–131.

23. Quétel, *History of Syphilis*, pp. 24–26; Jon Arrizabalaga, "Medical Responses to the 'French Disease' in Europe at the Turn of the Sixteenth Century," in Siena, *Sins of the Flesh*, pp. 33–55.

24. Quétel, *History of Syphilis*, pp. 53–54; Arrizabalaga et al., *The Great Pox*, pp. 50–52.

25. Peter Lewis Allen, *The Wages of Sin: Sex and Disease, Past and Present* (Chicago: University of Chicago Press, 2000), p. 42.

26. Quétel, *History of Syphilis*, p. 74

27. Arrizabalaga et al., *The Great Pox*, p. 123.

28. Mary Spongberg, *Feminizing Venereal Disease: The Body of the Prostitute in Nineteenth-Century Medical Discourse* (New York: New York University Press, 1997), pp. 1–6 (quotation on p. 3).

29. Ibid., pp. 2–3.

30. Ibid., p. 1.

31. Laura J. McGough, "Quarantining Beauty: The French Disease in Early Modern Venice," in Siena, *Sins of the Flesh*, pp. 211–237.

32. Vern L. Bullough, *The History of Prostitution* (New Hyde Park, NY: University Books, 1964), pp. 134–169.

33. Spongberg, *Feminizing Venereal Disease*, p. 6

34. Ibid., p. 10; John D'Emilio and Estelle B. Freedman, *Intimate Matters: A History of Sexuality in America*, 2nd ed. (Chicago: University of Chicago Press, 1997), p. 140; Annet Mooij, *Out of Otherness: Characters and Narrators in the Dutch Venereal Disease Debates 1850–1990* (Amsterdam: Editions Rodopi, 1998), pp. 32–34.

35. Quétel, *History of Syphilis*, p. 66; Arrizabalaga et al., *The Great Pox*, p. 129.

36. McGough, "Quarantining Beauty."

37. Sponberg, *Feminizing Venereal Disease*, pp. 36–37, 63.

38. Bruno P. F. Wanrooij, "'The Thorns of Love': Sexuality, Syphilis and Social Control in Modern Italy," in *Sex, Sin and Suffering: Venereal Disease and European Society Since 1870*, eds. Roger Davidson and Lesley A. Hall (London: Routledge, 2001), pp. 137–159 (quotation on p. 138).

39. Quétel, *History of Syphilis*, pp. 214–215.

40. Mooij, *Out of Otherness*, pp. 44–55.

41. Paula Bartley, *Prostitution: Prevention and Reform in England, 1860–1914* (London: Routledge, 2000), p. 12; Andrew Aisenberg, "Syphilis and Prostitution: A Regulatory Couplet in Nineteenth-Century France," in Davidson and Hall, *Sex, Sin and Suffering*, pp. 15–28.

42. Bullough, *History of Prostitution*, p. 172.

43. Arrizabalaga, "Medical Responses," p. 44; Barbara J. Dunlap, "The Problem of Syphilitic Children in Eighteenth-Century France and England," in Siena, *Sins of the Flesh*, pp. 114–127; David I. Kertzer, *Amalia's Tale: A Poor Peasant, an Ambitious Attorney, and a Fight for Justice* (Boston, MA: Houghton Mifflin Company, 2008), pp. 34–35.

44. Quetel, *History of Syphilis*, pp. 165–170, 250; Dunlap, "The Problem," p. 115.

45. Quoted (in English translation) from Quetel, *History of Syphilis*, p. 167.

46. Ibid., p. 250; Rosebury, *Microbes and Morals*, pp. 78–79.

47. Dunlap, "The Problem," pp. 118–121; Quetel, *History of Syphilis*, pp. 103–105

48. W. T. Watson, "Wet Nursing of Foundlings. A Pernicious Practice," *The Medico-Pharmaceutical Critic and Guide*, 7 (1906): 55–57 (quotations on. pp. 55–56).

49. Kertzer, *Amalia's Tale*.

50. Arrizabalaga et al., *The Great Pox*, p. 18.

51. Rosebury, *Microbes and Morals*, pp. 29–36; Quétel, *History of Syphilis*, pp. 52–53.

52. Quoted (in English translation) from Rosebury, *Microbes and Morals*, p. 33.

53. Stephen Jay Gould, "Syphilis and the Shepherd of Atlantis," *Natural History* 109 (October 2000): 38–42, 74–82.

54. Ibid.; Quétel, *History of Syphilis*, pp. 52–53; Arrizabalaga et al., *The Great Pox*, pp. 244–251.

55. Quétel, *History of Syphilis*, p. 53; Rosebury, *Microbes and Morals*, p. 29.

56. Deborah Hayden, *Pox: Genius, Madness, and the Mysteries of Syphilis* (New York: Basic Books, 2003).

57. Kevin Siena, "The Clean and the Foul: Paupers and the Pox in London Hospitals, c. 1550–c. 1700," in Siena, *Sins of the Flesh*, pp. 261–284.

58. Quétel, *History of Syphilis*, p. 23.

59. Arrizabalaga, et al., *The Great Pox*, pp. 29–30.

60. Quétel, *History of Syphilis*, pp. 30–32, 84; Owsei Temkin, "Therapeutic Trends and the Treatment of Syphilis before 1900," *Bulletin of the History of Medicine* 29 (1955): 309–316.

61. Quétel, *History of Syphilis*, pp. 85–86.

62. Hayden, *Pox*, pp. 48–49.

63. Quétel, *History of Syphilis*, pp. 27–30; Arrizabalaga et al., *The Great Pox*, pp. 99–103.

64. Watts, *Epidemics*, p. 130.

65. Quétel, *History of Syphilis*, pp. 63, 83–86, 116–117.

66. On the history of germ theory, see Gerald L. Geison, *The Private Science of Louis Pasteur* (Princeton, NJ: Princeton University Press, 1995); Nancy Tomes, *The Gospel of Germs: Men, Women, and the Microbe in American Life* (Cambridge, MA: Harvard University Press, 1998); Thomas Brock, *Robert Koch: A Life in Bacteriology and Medicine* (Madison, WI: Science Tech, 1988).

67. The literature on the history of smallpox and vaccination is extensive. For general overviews, see, for example, Donald R. Hopkins, *Princes and Peasants: Smallpox in History* (Chicago: University of Chicago Press, 1983); Jennifer Lee Carrell, *The Speckled Monster: A Historical Tale of Battling Smallpox* (New York: Dutton, 2003); Jonathan B. Tucker, *Scourge: The Once and Future Threat of Smallpox* (New York: Atlantic Monthly Press, 2001).

68. On the history of syphilization, see Joan Sherwood, "Syphilization: Human Experimentation in the Search for a Syphilis Vaccine in the Nineteenth Century," *Bulletin of the History of*

Medicine 54 (1999): 364–386; Alex Dracobly, "Ethics and Experimentation on Human Subjects in Mid-Nineteenth-Century France: The Story of the 1859 Syphilis Experiments," *Bulletin of the History of Medicine* 77 (2003): 332–366; Donald S. Burke, "Joseph-Alexandre Auzias-Turenne, Louis Pasteur, and Early Concepts of Virulence, Attenuation, and Vaccination," *Perspectives in Biology and Medicine* 39 (1996): 171–186; Stian E. Erichsen, "Auzias-Turenne's Syphilization Method in Norway: An Unsuccessful Attempt at Biologic Syphilis Therapy in the Middle of the Last Century," *American Journal of Syphilis, Gonorrhea, and Venereal Diseases* 35 (1951): 42–52.

69. Susan Lederer, *Subjected to Science: Human Experimentation in America before the Second World War* (Baltimore, MD: Johns Hopkins University Press, 1995), pp. 17–18; Jonathan D. Moreno, *Undue Risk: Secret State Experiments on Humans* (New York: Routledge, 2001), p. 20.

70. Richard M. Krause, "Metchnikoff and Syphilis Research during a Decade of Discovery, 1900–1910," *ASM News* 62 (1996): 307–310.

71. Quétel, *History of Syphilis*, pp. 140–141; Hayden, *Pox*, pp. 24–25.

72. Hayden, *Pox*, p. 49; Rosebury, *Microbes and Morals*, pp. 200–201.

73. John Parascandola, "The Theoretical Basis of Paul Ehrlich's Chemotherapy," *Journal of the History of Medicine* 36 (1981): 19–43.

CHAPTER TWO

1. Noble David Cook, *Born to Die: Disease and New World Conquest, 1492–1650* (Cambridge: Cambridge University Press, 1998), pp. 41–42.

2. Guenter B. Risse, "Medicine in New Spain," in *Medicine in the New World: New Spain, New France, and New England*, ed. Ronald L. Numbers (Knoxville, TN: University of Tennessee Press, 1987), pp. 12–63, 39–40.

3. Boyce Rensberger, "Colonial Remains Reclassified as African American," *Washington Post*, April 24, 1997, p. A3; Douglas W. Owsley, "Lessons from the Past," *CRM Online* 22 (1) (1999): 17–18, http://crm.cr.nps.gov.

4. John Duffy, *Epidemics in Colonial America* (Baton Rouge, LA: Louisiana State University Press, 1953), p. 233.

5. Carl Bridenbaugh, *Cities in the Wilderness: The First Century of Urban Life in America 1625–1742* (New York: Alfred A. Knopf, 1960), pp. 71–72, 226.

6. Duffy, *Epidemics*, pp. 33–34; Richard Harrison Shryock, *Medicine and Society in America, 1660–1860* (New York: New York University Press, 1960), pp. 92–93.

7. Richard Godbeer, *Sexual Revolution in Early America* (Baltimore, MD: Johns Hopkins University Press, 2002), p. 195.

8. Godbeer, *Sexual*, p. 179; John Duffy, *The Rudolph Matas History of Medicine in Louisiana*, Vol. 1 (Baton Rouge, LA: Louisiana State University Press, 1958), p. 39.

9. James Axtell, *The European and the Indian: Essays in the Ethnohistory of Colonial North America* (Oxford: Oxford University Press, 1981), pp. 154–155.

10. Alan Taylor, *American Colonies* (New York, Viking Penguin, 2001), pp. 460–466.

11. Quincy D. Newell, "'The Indians Generally Love Their Wives and Children': Native American Marriage and Sexual Practices in Missions San Francisco, Santa Clara, and San José," *The Catholic Historical Review* 91 (2005): 60–82, 76.

12. Colin G. Calloway, *The World Turned Upside Down: Indian Voices from Early America* (Boston, MA: St. Martin's Press, 1994), p. 2.

13. Duffy, *The Rudolph Matas History of Medicine in Louisiana*, pp. 39–40; Calloway, *World*, p. 4; Francis Parkman, *The Conspiracy of Pontiac and the Indian War after the Conquest of Canada* (Boston, MA: Little, Brown, 1886); "Jeffrey Amherst and the Smallpox Blankets," http://www.nativeweb.org/pages/legal/amherst/lord_jeff.html.

14. Todd L. Savitt, *Medicine and Slavery: The Diseases and Health Care of Blacks in Antebellum Virginia* (Urbana, IL: University of Illinois Press, 1978), pp. 77–78; John D'Emilio and Estelle B. Freedman, *Intimate Matters: A History of Sexuality in America*, 2nd ed. (Chicago: University of Chicago Press, 1997), pp. 12–14, 101–102; Godbeer, *Sexual Revolution*, pp. 216–223.

15. D'Emilio and Freedman, *Intimate Matters*, p. 12; David Lindsay, *Mayflower Bastard: A Stranger among the Pilgrims* (New York: St. Martin's Press, 2002), pp. 138–139.

16. Duffy, *Epidemics*, pp. 235–236.

17. Godbeer, *Sexual Revolution*, pp. 301–319; Oscar Reiss, *Medicine and the American Revolution* (Jefferson, NC: McFarland and Company, 1998), p. 156.

18. Reiss, *Medicine*, p. 162.

19. Mary C. Gillett, *The Army Medical Department 1775–1818* (Washington, DC: Center of Military History, United States Army, 1981), pp. 96–125; Reiss, *Medicine*, p. 163.

20. Gillett, *Army Medical Department 1775–1818*, pp. 5, 39.

21. Gerald N. Grob, *The Deadly Truth: A History of Disease in America* (Cambridge, MA: Harvard University Press, 2002), p. 197.

22. Duffy, *The Rudolph Matas History of Medicine in Louisiana*, pp. 287–288; "Venereal Disease," *Aurora General Advertiser*, July 21, 1797, p. 1.

23. John Duffy, *A History of Public Health in New York City, 1625–1868* (New York: Russell Sage Foundation, 1968), p. 265; John Duffy, "The Physician as a Moral Force in American History," in *New Knowledge in the Biomedical Sciences: Some Moral Implications of Its Acquisition, Possession, and Use*, eds. William B. Bondeson, H. Tristram Engelhardt, Jr., Stuart F. Spicker, and Joseph M. White (Dordrecht, Holland: D. Reidel Publishing, 1982), pp. 3–21, 11.

24. Thomas P. Lowry, *Venereal Disease and the Lewis and Clark Expedition* (Lincoln, NE: University of Nebraska Press, 2004), pp. 28–29.

25. Ibid., pp. 33–34.

26. Ibid., pp. 75–76.

27. Ibid., pp. 74–79.

28. Ibid., 82–83.

29. Ibid., pp. 93–101.

30. Ibid., p. 101.

31. Rudolph H. Kampmeier, "Venereal Disease in the United States Army: 1775–1900," *Sexually Transmitted Diseases* 9 (1982): 100–103; Gillett, *Army Medical Department 1775–1818*, p. 195.

32. Mary C. Gillett, *The Army Medical Department 1818–1865* (Washington, DC: Center of Military History, United States Army, 1987), pp. 88, 119.

33. D'Emilio and Freedman, *Intimate Matters*, pp. 130–134.

34. Ibid., pp. 134–135; Volney Steele, *Bleed, Blister, and Purge: A History of Medicine on the American Frontier* (Missoula, MT: Mountain Press, 2005), pp. 91–92.

35. Duffy, "Physician as a Moral Force," p. 11; Duffy, *Public Health*, pp. 265, 486–487; Francis R. Packard, *History of Medicine in the United States*, Vol. 1 (New York: Hoeber, 1931), p. 268.

36. D'Emilio and Freedman, *Intimate Matters*, p. 134.

37. Lawrence R. Murphy, "The Enemy among Us: Venereal Disease among Union Soldiers in the Far West, 1861–1865," *Civil War History* 31 (1985): 257–269, 258–259; James Boyd Jones, Jr., "A Tale of Two Cities: The Hidden Battle against Venereal Disease in Civil War Nashville and Memphis," *Civil War History* 31 (1985): 270–276, 271; Thomas P. Lowry, *The Story the Soldiers Wouldn't Tell: Sex in the Civil War* (Mechanicsburg, PA: Stackpole Books, 1994), pp. 105–107; H. H. Cunningham, *Doctors in Gray: The Confederate Medical Service*, 2nd ed. (Baton Rouge, LA: Louisiana State University Press, 1960), pp. 210–211.

38. Murphy, "Enemy among Us," pp. 259–265.

39. Murphy, "Enemy among Us," pp. 257–258; Jones, "Tale of Two Cities," pp. 273–274.

40. Jones, "Tale of Two Cities," pp. 270–276.

41. Lowry, *Story the Soldiers*, pp. 105–106.

42. Anne M. Butler, *Daughters of Joy, Sisters of Misery: Prostitutes in the American West, 1865–1890* (Urbana, IL: University of Illinois Press, 1985), pp. 9–13.

43. John C. Burnham, "Medical Inspection of Prostitutes in America in the Nineteenth Century: The St. Louis Experiment and Its Sequel," *Bulletin of the History of Medicine* 45 (1971): 203–218.

44. Ibid., p. 206.

45. Ibid., pp. 207–209 (quotation on p. 209); Duffy, "Physician as a Moral Force," p. 11.

46. Dorothy Porter, *Health, Civilization and the State: A History of Public Health from Ancient to Modern Times* (London: Routledge, 1999), pp. 155–159; John Duffy, *The Sanitarians: A History of American Public Health* (Urbana, IL: University of Illinois Press, 1992), pp. 130–132; Fitzhugh Mullan, *Plagues and Politics: The Story of the United States Public Health Service* (New York: Basic Books, 1989), pp. 14–25.

47. S. D. Gross, "Syphilis in Its Relation to the National Health," *Transactions of the American Medical Association* 25 (1874): 249–292.

48. Burnham, "Medical Inspection," p. 211.

49. Albert L. Gihon, *Report of the Committee on the Prevention of Venereal Diseases* (Boston, MA: Franklin Press: Rand, Avery, and Company, 1881).

50. Ibid., pp. 5–9.

51. Ibid., p. 13.

52. Ibid., p. 11.

53. Ibid., pp. 14–18 (quotation on pp. 15–16).

54. Burnham, "Medical Inspection," p. 213.

55. Ibid., pp. 213–215.

56. D'Emilio and Freedman, *Intimate Matters*, pp. 148–150 (quotation on pp. 149–150).

57. Aaron M. Powell, *State Regulation of Vice: Regulation Efforts in America, The Geneva Congress* (New York: Wood and Holbrook, 1878).

58. Ibid., p. 24.

59. Allan M. Brandt, *No Magic Bullet: A Social History of Venereal Disease in the United States Since 1880*, expanded edition (Oxford: Oxford University Press, 1987), pp. 7–23.

60. Daniel J. Kevles, *In the Name of Eugenics: Genetics and the Uses of Human Heredity* (Cambridge, MA: Harvard University Press, 1995); Alexandra Minna Stern, *Eugenic Nation: Faults and Frontiers of Better Breeding in Modern America* (Berkeley, CA: University of California Press, 2005).

61. Brandt, *No Magic Bullet*, p. 9.

62. Ibid., p. 14.

63. Ibid., pp. 14–16 (quotation on p. 14).

64. Ibid., pp. 20–21; D'Emilio and Freedman, *Intimate Matters*, p. 209; Amy L. Fairchild, *Science at the Borders: Immigrant Medical Inspection and the Shaping of the Modern Industrial Labor Force* (Baltimore, MD: Johns Hopkins University Press, 2003), pp. 172–173; Alan M. Kraut, *Silent Travelers: Germs, Genes, and the "Immigrant Menace"* (New York: Basic Books, 1994), p. 123.

65. James H. Jones, *Bad Blood: The Tuskegee Syphilis Experiment*, expanded edition (New York: The Free Press, 1993), pp. 23–24.

66. Ibid., p. 24.

67. John S. Haller, Jr., *Outcasts from Evolution: Scientific Attitudes of Racial Inferiority 1859–1900*, new edition (Carbondale, IL: Southern Illinois University Press, 1995), pp. 49–60.

68. Jones, *Bad Blood*, pp. 24–27 (quotation on p. 27).

69. H. H. Hazen, "Syphilis in the American Negro," *Journal of the American Medical Association* 63 (1914): 463–466 (quotation on p. 463).

70. Kenneth M. Lynch, B. Kater McInnes, and G. Fleming McInnes, "Concerning Syphilis in the American Negro," *Southern Medical Journal* 8 (1915): 450–456 (quotation on p. 452).

71. Thomas W. Murrell, "Syphilis and the American Negro: A Medico-Sociologic Study," *Journal of the American Medical Association* 54 (1910): 846–849 (quotation is on p. 847).

72. Brandt, *No Magic Bullet*, pp. 12–13.

73. D'Emilio and Freedman, *Intimate Matters*, p. 203.

74. Paul S. Boyer, ed., *The Oxford Companion to United States History* (Oxford: Oxford University Press, 2001), pp. 623–624 (quotation on p. 623).

75. Nancy R. Bristow, *Making Men Moral: Social Engineering during the Great War* (New York: New York University Press, 1996), pp. 16–17, 25–26, 80–81.

76. D'Emilio and Freedman, *Intimate Matters*, pp. 203–204 (quotation on p. 204).

77. Ibid., pp. 204–205; Brandt, *No Magic Bullet*, pp. 12–17; David Klaasen and Kay Flaminio, *Celebrating 80 Years: American Social Health Association* (Research Triangle Park, NC: American Social Health Association, 1994), pp. 2–3.

78. Prince A. Morrow, "The Sanitary Supervision of Prostitutes," *Interstate Medical Journal* 18 (1911): 98–108 (quotation on p. 105).

79. Brandt, *No Magic Bullet*, pp. 23–24.

80. Prince Morrow to Mary Cobb, September 13, 1909, ASHA Records, box 1, folder 4.

81. Klaasen and Flaminio, *Celebrating*, pp. 2–3; Brandt, *No Magic Bullet*, pp. 24–25.

82. Brandt, *No Magic Bullet*, p. 34.

83. Bullough, *History of Prostitution*, pp. 173–174; Mary E. Odem, *Delinquent Daughters: Protecting and Policing Adolescent Female Sexuality in the United States, 1885–1920* (Chapel Hill, NC: University of North Carolina Press, 1995), p. 97.

84. Ruth Rosen, *The Lost Sisterhood: Prostitution in America, 1900–1918* (Baltimore, MD: Johns Hopkins University Press, 1982), p. 118.

85. Ibid., pp. 112–135; Bullough, *History of Prostitution*, p. 183.

86. Brandt, *No Magic Bullet*, pp. 36–37.

87. Ibid., p. 38; Klaasen and Flaminio, *Celebrating*, pp. 3–5.

88. William F. Snow, "Progress, 1900–1915," *Social Hygiene* 2 (1916): 37–47 (quotation on p. 37).

89. Brandt, *No Magic Bullet*, p. 41.

90. Ibid., pp. 41–43.

91. Ibid., p. 46.

CHAPTER THREE

1. Allan M. Brandt, *No Magic Bullet: A Social History of Venereal Disease in the United States Since 1880*, expanded edition (Oxford: Oxford University Press, 1987), pp. 53–56; Linda Sharon Janke, "Prisoners of War: Sexuality, Venereal Disease, and Women's Incarceration during World War I," Ph.D. dissertation, Binghamton University, State University of New York, 2006, pp. 1–3.

2. [Raymond Fosdick], untitled 5-page typescript, no date, CTCA records, Reports Relating to Training Camp Activities, 1917 (entry 395), box 1, Alabama 1.3 folder.

3. Brandt, *No Magic Bullet*, pp. 54–55.

4. Ibid., pp. 54–56; Janke, "Prisoners of War," pp. 2–3.

5. Brandt, *No Magic Bullet*, p. 56.

6. Ibid., p. 57; Nancy R. Bristow, *Making Men Moral: Social Engineering during the Great War* (New York: New York University Press, 1996), pp. 1–3.

7. M. J. Exner to Frank Ober, May 23, 1917, CTCA Records, Reports on Training Camp Activities, 1917 (entry 395), box 1, Alabama 6 folder; Brandt, *No Magic Bullet*, pp. 56–59.

8. Brandt, *No Magic Bullet*, pp. 59–60; Bristow, *Making Men Moral*, pp. 7–8; Janke, "Prisoners of War," pp. 3–4; Nancy Moore Rockafellar, "Making the World Safe for the Soldiers of Democracy: Patriotism, Public Health and Venereal Disease Control on the West Coast, 1910–1919," Ph.D. dissertation, University of Washington, 1990, pp. 194–195.

9. Rockafellar, "Making the World Safe," pp. 191–192.

10. Brandt, *No Magic Bullet*, pp. 58–59; minutes of meetings of May 26 and June 28, 1917, CTCA Records, Minutes (entry 403), box 02.

11. Newton D. Baker to Governors of all States and Chairmen of State Councils of Defense, May 26, 1917, CCCCVD Records, box 437.

12. Executive Secretary, CCCCVD to Jeanette Rankin, January 29, 1918, CCCCVD Records, box 440.

13. Michael Imber, "The First World War, Sex Education, and the American Social Hygiene Association's Campaign Against Venereal Disease," *Journal of Educational Administration and History* 16 (1984): 47–56.

14. Brandt, *No Magic Bullet*, p. 53.

15. 5. Quoted from Imber, "The First World War," p. 49 and Janke, "Prisoners of War," p. 46, respectively.

16. Brandt, *No Magic Bullet*, pp. 110–116.

17. George Walker, *Venereal Disease in the American Expeditionary Forces* (Baltimore, MD: Medical Standard Book Company, 1922); Brandt, *No Magic Bullet*, pp. 96–121.

18. [Raymond Fosdick], untitled 5-page typescript, no date, CTCA records.

19. The War Department, *Commission on Training Camp Activities* (Washington, DC: War Department, no date), pp. 3–4 (quotations on p. 4). There is a copy of this booklet in the National Archives Library, College Park, MD.

20. Ibid., pp. 4–6.

21. Edward H. Beardsley, "Allied against Sin: American and British Responses to Venereal Disease in World War I," *Medical History* 20 (1976): 189–202 (the quotation is on p. 193).

22. Minutes of meeting, April 26, 1917, CTCA Records, Minutes (entry 403), box 02.

23. Bristow, *Making Men Moral*, p. 241.

24. Newton D. Baker to "My Dear Sir," August 10, 1917, ASHA Records, box 19, folder 2.

25. Brandt, *No Magic Bullet*, pp. 73–77; Raymond Fosdick to William Martin, July 7, 1917, CTCA records, Reports Relating to Training Camp Activities, 1917 (entry 395), box 1, Alabama 1.3 folder.

26. Bascom Johnson, "Preliminary Report on Moral Conditions in California, June 20 to July 21st, 1917," 14-page typescript; Bascom Johnson, "Preliminary Report on Moral Conditions Surrounding the Military Camp at Linda Vista and the Naval Training Station at San Diego, California, July 17–19, 1917," 10-page typescript, CTCA records, Reports Relating to Training Camp Activities, 1917 (entry 395), box 5, California (San Diego) folder.

27. Bristow, *Making Men Moral*, p. 112.

28. Ibid., pp. 113–114.

29. Mary E. Odem, *Delinquent Daughters: Protecting and Policing Adolescent Female Sexuality in the United States, 1885–1920* (Chapel Hill, NC: University of North Carolina Press, 1995); Ruth M. Alexander, *The "Girl Problem": Female Sexual Delinquency in New York, 1900–1930* (Ithaca, NY: Cornell University Press, 1995); Kathy Peiss, "'Charity Girls' and City Pleasures: Historical Notes on Working Class Sexuality," in *Powers of Desire: The Politics of Sexuality*, eds. Ann Snitow, Christine Stansell, and Sharon Thompson (New York: Monthly Review Press, 1983), pp. 74–87.

30. Bristow, *Making Men Moral*, p. 117.

31. Ibid., pp. 114–116; Janke, "Prisoners of War," pp. 71–87.

32. Janke, "Prisoners of War," pp. 68–70, 97.

33. Ibid., p. 69.

34. Ibid., pp. 100–111; Bristow, *Making Men Moral*, pp. 125–126.

35. Janke, "Prisoners of War," p. 115.

36. Brandt, *No Magic Bullet*, pp. 88–89; Mary Marcy Dietzler, *Detention Houses and Reformatories as Protective Social Agencies in the Campaign of the United States Government against Venereal Disease* (Washington, DC: Government Printing Office, 1922), pp. 29, 33, 69.

37. Brandt, *No Magic Bullet*, p. 234 (fn. 118); Janke, "Prisoners of War," p. 7; Bristow, *Making Men Moral*, p. 129.

38. Brandt, *No Magic Bullet*, p. 85; Janke, "Prisoners of War," pp. 299–319.

39. David J. Pivar, *Purity and Hygiene: Women, Prostitution, and the "American Plan," 1900–1930* (Westport, CT: Greenwood Press, 2002), p. 211.

40. Torald Sollmann, *A Manual of Pharmacology and Its Applications to Therapeutics and Toxicology* (Philadelphia, PA: W.B. Saunders, 1917), pp. 748–755.

41. Brandt, *No Magic Bullet*, p. 46.

42. Rockafellar, "Making the World Safe," p. 348.

43. Michael Lowenthal, *Charity Girl* (Boston, MA: Houghton Mifflin, 2007). The author's note is on pp. 319–320. The quotation about Frieda is from the dust jacket.

44. Dietzler, *Detention Houses*.

45. Ibid., p. 75; Brandt, *No Magic Bullet*, p. 90.

46. Dietzler, *Detention Houses*, pp. 91–95.

47. Brandt, *No Magic Bullet*, p. 92.

48. Bristow, *Making Men Moral*, p. 135; Brandt, *No Magic Bullet*, p. 73; Sue Sun Yom, "Sex and the American Soldier: Military Cinema and the War on Venereal Disease, 1918–1969," Ph.D. dissertation, University of Pennsylvania, 2003, p. 16.

49. Beardsley, "Allied against Sin," p. 194.

50. Thomas A. Storey, "Letter of Transmittal," in Dietzler, *Detention Houses*, pp. 1–2 (quotation on p. 2).

51. Sarah Mercer Judson, "'Leisure is a Foe to Any Man': The Pleasures and Dangers of Leisure in Atlanta during World War I," *Journal of Women's History* 15 (2003): 92–115 (quotation on p. 98).

52. Janke, "Prisoners of War," pp. 57–58; Brandt, *No Magic Bullet*, p. 58; Barbara Meil Hobson, *Uneasy Virtue: The Politics of Prostitution and the American Reform Tradition* (New York: Basic Books, 1987), pp. 180–181.

53. Sample pamphlet and poster formats attached to letter from William H. Zinsser, Social Hygiene Division, CTCA, to Managing Executive, Loet Schmutt, Inc., December 24, 1918, PHS VD Division Records, 405.1, box 213.

54. Bristow, *Making Men Moral*, pp.130–136; Hobson, *Uneasy Virtue*, pp. 180–181; Brandt, *No Magic Bullet*, p. 86.

55. Hobson, *Uneasy Virtue*; Odem, *Delinquent Daughters*; Alexander, *The Girl Problem*; Janke, "Prisoners of War."

56. Janke, "Prisoners of War," pp. 131–137; Brandt, *No Magic Bullet*, p. 86; Allison French to Bascom Johnson, September 6, 1917, CTCA Records, Reports Relating to Training Camp Activities, 1917 (entry 395), box 5, California (December 1917) folder.

57. Bristow, *Making Men Moral*, pp. 36–45, 56–59; Brandt, *No Magic Bullet*, pp. 60–61.

58. Weldon B. Durham, *Liberty Theatres of the United States Army, 1917–1919* (Jefferson, NC: McFarland, 2006).

59. Bristow, *Making Men Moral*, pp. 59–64, 79–88; Judson, "Leisure is a Foe."

60. Brandt, *No Magic Bullet*, pp. 61–63.

61. "Notes on the History of the Social Hygiene Division. Commission on Training Camp Activities. War and Navy Departments," 10-page document, handwritten date of October 7, 1919, ASHA Records, box 131, folder 3.

62. "Syllabus for Use in Lectures on Sex Hygiene and Venereal Diseases to Men in Uniform and in Class 1," CCTA, May 1918, ASHA Records, box 131, folder 6 (quotations on p. 3); "Syllabus Accredited for Use in Official Supplementary Lectures on Sex Hygiene and Venereal Diseases Approved by the Surgeon General, USN," Navy CCTA, February 1918 (unpaginated), CCTA Records, General Correspondence, 1917–1921 (entry 393), box 54, items 26241–26242.

63. Ibid.

64. Yom, "Sex and the American Soldier," pp. 26–28; Brandt, *No Magic Bullet*, pp. 68–69; Robert Eberwein, *Sex Ed: Film, Video, and the Framework of Desire* (New Brunswick, NJ: Rutgers University Press, 1999), pp. 21–31.

65. Yom, "Sex and the American Soldier," p. 28.

66. William H. Zinsser to Managing Executive, Loet Schmutt, Inc., December 24, 1918; "Outline of Plan of the War Department Commission on Training Camp Activities for Combating Venereal Disease in Industrial Plants," one-page flyer, ASHA Records, box 131, folder 3; Bristow, *Making Men Moral*, p. 65.

67. Form letter signed by Katharine Bement Davis, no date, ASHA Records, box 131, folder 8.

68. Eberwein, *Sex Ed*, pp. 31–33; Yom, "Sex and the American Soldier," pp. 31–35 (quotation on p. 31); Brandt, *No Magic Bullet*, p. 83.

69. Bristow, *Making Men Moral*, p. 65.

70. Ibid., pp. 137–138.

71. Ibid., pp. 141–144; Judson, "Leisure is a Foe," pp. 106–107.

72. Raymond Fosdick to Newton D. Baker, October 10, 1917, CTCA Records, Reports Relating to Training Camp Activities, 1917 (entry 395), box 1, Alabama 3 folder.

73. Bristow, *Making Men Moral*, pp. 146–157, 164–169; P. Robertson and F.B. Barnes to Raymond Fosdick, October 20, 1917, CTCA Records, General Correspondence, 1917–1921 (entry 393), box 55, Kansas (Fort Riley) folder.

74. Bristow, *Making Men Moral*, pp. 157–158.

75. Ibid., p. 159; Raymond Fosdick to George A. Nesbitt, September 14, 1917 and Executive Secretary to Reverends Wood, Pierce and Wilfley, August 27, 1917, CTCA Records, Reports on Training Camp Activities, 1917 (entry 395), box 5, DC folder.

76. Report by J.S., September 14, 1917, attached to letter from John F. Luhrs to Raymond Fosdick, September 18, 1917, CTCA Records, Reports on Training Camp Activities, 1917 (entry 395), box 5, DC folder.

77. Janke, "Prisoners of War," pp. 127–129; Bristow, *Making Men Moral*, p. 162.

78. Brandt, *No Magic Bullet*, pp. 116–117; Toni P. Miles and David McBride, "World War I Origins of the Syphilis Epidemic among 20th Century Black Americans: A Biohistorical Analysis," *Social Science & Medicine* 45 (1997): 61–69.

79. Fitzhugh Mullan, *Plagues and Politics: The Story of the United States Public Health Service* (New York: Basic Books, 1989); Ralph Chester Williams, *The United States Public Health Service, 1798–1950* (Washington, DC: Commissioned Officers Association of the United States Public Health Service, 1951).

80. Ibid.; "Venereal Disease Control," 5-page typescript, no date, PHS VD Division Records, 308.2, box 183.

81. Williams, *Public Health Service*, pp. 590–592; "Summary of Venereal Disease Work of the U.S. Public Health Service from January 1, 1918 to June 30, 1924," 62-page typescript, 1925, PHS VD Division Records, 308.2, box 183.

CHAPTER FOUR

1. Rupert Blue to Herbert D. Brown, December 30, 1918, PHS VD Division Records, 308, box 182.

2. Nancy R. Bristow, *Making Men Moral: Social Engineering during the Great War* (New York: New York University Press, 1996), pp. 180–184.

3. Allan M. Brandt, *No Magic Bullet: A Social History of Venereal Disease in the United States Since 1880*, expanded edition (Oxford: Oxford University Press, 1987), pp. 122–123 (quotations on p. 122).

4. Ibid., pp. 124–125.

5. Walter Clarke to Ray Lyman Wilbur, August 16, 1940, ASHA Records, box 117, folder 4.

6. Brandt, *No Magic Bullet*, pp. 157–158 (quotations on p. 158).

7. Alexandra M. Lord, "Models of Masculinity: Sex Education, the United States Public Health Service, and the YMCA, 1919–1924," *Journal of the History of Medicine* 58 (2003): 123–152 (quotation on p. 133).

8. Alexandra M. Lord, "'Naturally Clean and Wholesome': Women, Sex Education, and the United States Public Health Service, 1918–1928," *Social History of Medicine* 17 (2004): 423–441.

9. Adolf Nichtenhauser, "A History of Motion Pictures in Medicine," unpublished typescript, ca. 1950, MS C 380, History of Medicine Division, National Library of Medicine, Bethesda, MD, II, 98–110; Martin S. Pernick, "Sex Education Films, U.S. Government," *Isis* 84 (1993): 766–768.

10. Nichtenhauser, "History of Motion Pictures," p. 125.

11. Thomas Parran, *Shadow on the Land: Syphilis* (New York: Reynal and Hitchcock, 1937), p. 85; James H. Jones, *Bad Blood: The Tuskegee Syphilis Experiment*, expanded edition (New York: The Free Press, 1993), p. 50.

12. Walter Clarke to Thomas Parran, May 10, 1940; Thomas Parran to Walter Clarke, May 15, 1940, ASHA Records, box 115, folder 1.

13. Brandt, *No Magic Bullet*, pp. 126–129 (quotation on pp. 128–129), 156.

14. William A. Snow to John D. Rockefeller, Jr., January 7, 1919 (quotation); John D. Rockefeller, Jr., to Edward L. Keyes, July 7, 1919, ASHA Records, box 25, folder 9.

15. "The American Social Hygiene Association: Special Bulletin for Members, October, 1925," 4-page typescript, ASHA Records, box 19, folder 6.

16. David Klaasen and Kay Flaminio, *Celebrating 80 Years: American Social Health Association* (Research Triangle Park, NC: American Social Health Association, 1994), pp. 9–10; Brandt, *No Magic Bullet*, p. 131.

17. "Damaged Lives: A Photoplay with a Purpose," brochure (New York: American Social Hygiene Association, no date), ASHA Records, box 69, folder 7.

18. Robert Eberwein, *Sex Ed: Film, Video, and the Framework of Desire* (New Brunswick, NJ: Rutgers University Press, 1999), pp. 36–39 (quotations on p. 38); Elizabeth Fee, "Sin vs. Science: Venereal Disease in Baltimore in the Twentieth Century," *Bulletin of the History of Medicine* 43 (1988): 141–164.

19. Susan Lederer, *Subjected to Science: Human Experimentation in America before the Second World War* (Baltimore, MD: Johns Hopkins University Press, 1995), pp. 82–87 (quotation on p. 82).

20. Ibid., pp. 95–100.

21. Janice Dickin McGinnis, "From Salvarsan to Penicillin: Medical Science and VD Control in Canada," in *Essays in the History of Canadian Medicine*, eds. Wendy Mitchinson and Janice Dicken McGinnis (Toronto: McClelland and Stewart, 1988), pp. 126–147; R. H. Kampmeier, "Syphilis Therapy: An Historical Perspective," *Journal of the American Venereal Disease Association* 3 (1976): 99–108; *Milestones in Venereal Disease Control: Highlights of a Half-Century* (Washington, DC: U.S. Department of Health, Education, and Welfare, 1957); Jay Casell, *The Secret Plague: Venereal Disease in Canada 1838–1939* (Toronto: University of Toronto Press, 1987), p. 56.

22. Jeffrey S. Sartin and Harold O. Perry, "From Mercury to Malaria to Penicillin: The History of the Treatment of Syphilis at the Mayo Clinic—1916–1955," *Journal of the American Academy of Dermatology* 32 (1995): 255–261.

23. *Nobel Lectures, Physiology or Medicine 1922–1941* (Amsterdam: Elsevier, 1965); Paul Weindling, "Julius Wagner-Jauregg," in *Nobel Laureates in Medicine or Physiology: A Biographical Dictionary*, eds. Daniel M. Fox, Marcia Meldrum, and Ira Rezak (New York: Garland Publishing, 1990), pp. 545–548; Sartin and Perry, "From Mercury"; Joel Braslow, "The Influence of a Biological Therapy on Physicians' Narratives and Interrogations: The Case of General Paralysis of the Insane and Malaria Fever Therapy, 1910–1950," *Bulletin of the History of Medicine* 70 (1996): 577–608.

24. Braslow, "The Influence," pp. 606–607.

25. Kampmeier, "Syphilis Therapy," p. 105; Louis Chargin and William Leifer, "Massive Dose Arsenotherapy of Early Syphilis by Intravenous 'Drip Method,'" *A. M. A. Archives of Dermatology* 73 (1956): 482–484; Harold Thomas Hyman, "Massive Arsenotherapy in Early Syphilis by the Continuous Intravenous Drip Method," *Archives of Dermatology and Syphilology* 42 (1940): 253–261; "Massive Arsenotherapy for Syphilis," *Journal of the American Medical Association* 126 (1944): 554–557.

26. James Harvey Young, *The Toadstool Millionaires: A Social History of Patent Medicines in America before Federal Regulation* (Princeton, NJ: Princeton University Press, 1961), pp. 58–66, 114–117.

27. Brooks McNamara, *Step Right Up: An Illustrated History of the American Medical Show* (Garden City, NY: Doubleday, 1976), p. 42.

28. James Harvey Young, *The Medical Messiahs: A Social History of Health Quackery in Twentieth-Century America* (Princeton, NJ: Princeton University Press, 1967), p. 84; Ruth deForest Lamb, *American Chamber of Horrors: The Truth about Food and Drugs* (New York: Farrar and Rinehart, 1936), p. 71; F. J. Cullan, "Federal Control of Venereal Disease Nostrums Through Proposed Legislation," *Journal of Social Hygiene* 19 (1933): 513–522.

29. Arthur Oslo, George E. Farrar, Jr., and Robertson Pratt, *Dispensatory of the United States of America 1960 Edition* (Philadelphia, PA: J. B. Lippincott, 1960), p. 1215; David M. R. Culbreth, *A Manual of Materia Medica and Pharmacology*, 6th ed. (Philadelphia, PA: Lea and Febiger, 1917), p. 121; Arthur R. Cushny, *A Textbook of Pharmacology and Therapeutics*, 3rd ed. (Philadelphia, PA: Lea Brothers, 1903), p. 355.

30. Young, *Toadstool Millionaires*, p. 168; Casell, *Secret Plague*, p. 63; Suzanne Poirier, *Chicago's War on Syphilis, 1937–1940: The Times, the Trib, and the Clap Doctor* (Urbana, IL: University of Illinois Press, 1995), pp. 61–63.

31. Cullan, "Federal Control," p. 519.

32. James Harvey Young, "Device Quackery in America," *Bulletin of the History of Medicine* 39 (1965): 154–162.

33. Parran, *Shadow*, p. 248.

34. W. C. Murphy to Thomas Parran, Jr., October 22, 1926, PHS VD Division Records, 308.2, box 183; Mark J. White to A. M. Stimson, October 2, 1923, PHS VD Division Records, 308.2, box 183; Brandt, *No Magic Bullet*, p. 131.

35. Murphy to Parran, October 22, 1926 (quotation); Edwina Walls, "Hot Springs Waters and the Treatment of Venereal Diseases: The U.S. Public Health Service Clinic and Camp Garraday," *Journal of the Arkansas Medical Society* 91 (1995): 430–437.

36. Brandt, *No Magic Bullet*, p. 131.

37. Poirier, *Chicago's War*, pp. 138–139; Jones, *Bad Blood*, pp. 30–44.

38. Jones, *Bad Blood*, pp. 52–55.

39. Ibid., pp. 58–60.

40. Ibid., pp. 61–90.

41. On the Tuskegee Syphilis Study, see Ibid.; Susan M. Reverby, ed., *Tuskegee's Truths: Rethinking the Tuskegee Syphilis Study* (Chapel Hill, NC: University of North Carolina Press, 2000); Allan M. Brandt, "Racism and Research: The Case of the Tuskegee Syphilis Experiment," *The Hastings Center Report* 8 (December 1978): 21–29; Thomas Benedek, "The 'Tuskegee Study' of Syphilis: Analysis of Moral versus Methodological Aspects," *Journal of Chronic Diseases* 31 (1978): 35–50; Stephen B. Thomas and Sandra Crouse Quinn, "The Tuskegee Syphilis Study, 1932–1972: Implications for HIV Education and AIDS Risk Education Programs in the Black Community," *American Journal of Public Health* 81 (1991): 1498–1505; Vanessa Northington Gamble, "Under the Shadow of Tuskegee: African Americans and Health Care," *American Journal of Public Health* 87 (1997): 1773–1787. All of the articles cited in this note are reprinted in Reverby, *Tuskegee's Truths*.

42. Jones, *Bad Blood*, pp. 91–94; R. A. Vonderlehr to the Surgeon General, July 10, 1933, PHS VD Division Records, 308.1, box 182.

43. Jones, *Bad Blood*, pp. 94–95.

44. Susan L. Smith, "Neither Victim nor Villain: Eunice Rivers and Public Health Work," *Journal of Women's History* 8 (1996): 95–113, reprinted in Reverby, *Tuskegee's Truths*, pp. 348–364.

45. Benedek, "Tuskegee Study;" Jones, *Bad Blood*, pp. 98–99, 116–119, 126–130 (quotation on p. 119).

46. Brandt, "Racism and Research."

47. Jones, *Bad Blood*, p. 173.

48. Pasquale J. Pesare, in "Transcript of Proceedings, Federal Security Agency, Public Health Service, Venereal Disease Control Field Staff Conference," Washington, DC, April 24, 1950, p. 181, CDC Records, Acc. 63A0314, "Venereal Disease Field Staff Conference."

49. Ibid., pp. 188–205.

50. Brandt, "Racism and Research"; "Selections from the Final Report of the Ad Hoc Tuskegee Syphilis Study Panel, Department of Health, Education, and Welfare, 1973," in Reverby, *Tuskegee's Truths*, pp. 157–181.

51. Susan E. Bell, "Events in the Tuskegee Syphilis Study: A Timeline," in Reverby, *Tuskegee's Truths*, pp. 34–38; "President William J. Clinton's Remarks: Remarks by the President in Apology for Study Done in Tuskegee," in Reverby, *Tuskegee's Truths*, pp. 574–577; Thomas and Quinn, "Tuskegee Syphilis Study."

52. Jones, *Bad Blood*, pp. 35, 171–172 (quotation on p. 172).

53. Ibid., p. 41.

54. Ibid., pp. 57, 88, 107, 123, 134 (quotation on p. 88).

55. Leroy E. Burney, "Control of Syphilis in a Southern Rural Area," *American Journal of Public Health* 29 (1939): 1006–1014 (quotations on pp. 1009 and 1014); John Parascandola, "Syphilis at the Cinema: Medicine and Morals in VD Films of the U.S. Public Health Service in World War II," in *Medicine's Moving Pictures: Medicine, Health, and Bodies in American Film and Television*, eds. Leslie J. Reagan, Nancy Tomes, and Paula A. Treichler (Rochester, NY: University of Rochester Press, 2007), pp. 71–92.

56. Parran, *Shadow*, pp. 175–177 (quotation on p. 175).

57. Lynne Page Snyder, "Thomas J. Parran, Jr.," in *Doctors, Nurses, and Medical Practitioners: A Bio-Bibliographic Sourcebook*, ed. Lois N. Magner (Westport, CT: Greenwood Press, 1997), pp. 209–215.

58. Jones, *Bad Blood*, p. 58.

59. J. L. Smith, "Roosevelt Asks Parran to Direct Bureau of Health," *Albany Knickerbocker*, February 20, 1930.

60. "Special Activities for Control of Syphilis," *Health News* 12(25) (published weekly by New York State Department of Health), June 24, 1935, pp. 97–98 (copy in Parran Papers, FF173).

61. "Talk Censored, Dr. Parran Quits Radio Council," *New York Herald Tribune*, November 21, 1934.

62. William F. Snow to William S. Paley, and William F. Snow to Robert A. Millikan, November 20, 1934; John L. Rice to William F. Snow, November 22, 1934, ASHA Records, box 70, folder 4.

63. M. H. Aylesworth to John L. Rice, November 22, 1934; G. W. Grignon to Hazel I. McCarthy, January 10, 1934, ASHA Records, box 70. folder 4.

64. Snyder, "Thomas J. Parran, Jr.," p. 211.

65. Brandt, *No Magic Bullet*, p. 138.

66. Parran, *Shadow*, pp. 89–110 (quotation on p. 97).

67. Ibid., p. vii.

68. Ibid., p. 296.

69. Ibid., pp. 276–277.

70. Thomas Parran, "Syphilis Can Be Stamped Out," *Readers Digest*, April 1937, pp. 21–25 (quotation on p. 25).

71. Parran, *Shadow*, pp. 204–206, 220–223, 276–277; Thomas Parran to George Healy, Jr., September 16, 1944, PHS Records, GCR, 1936-44, 0425, 1944 folder.

72. "Great Pox," *Time*, October 26, 1936; Brandt, *No Magic Bullet*, p. 141.

73. "Venereal Disease Campaign," *Time*, January 11, 1937; Brandt, *No Magic Bullet*, p. 143 (quotation from Roosevelt appears in both sources).

74. "Asks Funds for War on Social Disease," *New York Times*, December 31, 1936; "Signs Bill for Fight on Venereal Disease," *New York Times*, May 26, 1938; "Millions v. Germs," *Time*, May 30, 1938; Brandt, *No Magic Bullet*, pp. 143–145.

75. Brandt, *No Magic Bullet*, pp. 144–147 (quotation on p. 147).

76. Ibid., pp. 147–150; George Gould, "Twenty Years' Progress in Social Hygiene Legislation," *Journal of Social Hygiene* 30 (1944): 456–471.

77. Brandt, *No Magic Bullet*, p. 151.

78. Poirier, *Chicago's War*, pp. 7–10, 14, 22, 30–31, 91–93.

79. Barbara Melosh, "The New Deal's Federal Theatre Project," *Medical Heritage* 2 (January/February 1986): 36–47; Barry Witham, *The Federal Theatre Project: A Case Study* (Cambridge: Cambridge University Press, 2003), pp. 113–120; Hallie Flanagan, *Arena: The Story of the Federal Theatre* (New York: Limelight Editions, 1969), p. 144.

CHAPTER FIVE

1. Richard B. Morris, ed., *Encyclopedia of American History*, updated and revised edition (New York: Harper and Row, 1965), pp. 363–365.

2. Ebbe Curtiss Hoff, ed., *Preventive Medicine in World War II*, Vol. 5 (Washington, DC: Office of the Surgeon General, Department of the Army, 1960), p. 140.

3. Ibid., Appendix B.

4. Ibid., pp. 142–143, Appendix C; Odin W. Anderson, *Syphilis and Society—Problems of Control in the United States, 1912–1964* (Chicago: Center for Health Administration Studies, Health Information Foundation, 1965), p. 13; Brandt, *No Magic Bullet*, p. 166.

5. Thomas Parran and Raymond Vonderlehr, *Plain Words about Venereal Disease* (New York: Reynal and Hitchcock, 1941), pp. 1 (quotation), 87–91; Hoff, *Preventive Medicine*, Vol. 8 (1976), pp. 61–62; Brandt, *No Magic Bullet*, p. 162; Thomas Parran to T. H. D. Griffitts, November 22, 1941, Pritchard Papers, box 3.

6. Brandt, *No Magic Bullet*, pp. 162–163

7. Hoff, *Preventive Medicine*, Vol. 8, p. 63.

8. Hoff, *Preventive Medicine*, Vol. 3, pp. 6–7.

9. Mattie E. Treadwell, *The Women's Army Corps* (Washington, DC: Center of Military History, United States Army, 1991), pp. 602–609.

10. Brandt, *No Magic Bullet*, p. 163

11. Meghan Kate Winchell, "Good Food, Good Fun, and Good Girls: USO Hostesses and World War Two," Ph.D. dissertation, University of Arizona, 2003, pp. 11–14; Marilyn E. Hegarty, *Victory Girls, Khaki-Wackies, and Patriotutes: The Regulation of Female Sexuality during World War II* (New York: New York University Press, 2008), pp. 1–8.

12. Winchell, "Good Food," pp. 22–25.

13. Granville W. Larimore and Thomas H. Sternberg, "Does Health Education Prevent Venereal Disease? The Army's Experience with 8,000,000 Men," *American Journal of Public Health* 35 (1945): 799–804 (quotation on p. 799).

14. Ibid., pp. 801–802 (quotations on p. 802).

15. Herb Friedman, "Venereal Disease Propaganda," http://www.psywarrior.com/PSYOPVD.html.

16. Robert Eberwein, *Sex Ed: Film, Video, and the Framework of Desire* (New Brunswick, NJ: Rutgers University Press, 1999), pp. 64–86.

17. Stan Lee and George Mair, *Excelsior! The Amazing Life of Stan Lee* (New York: Simon and Schuster, 2002), p. 45 (quotation); Friedman, "Venereal Disease Propaganda."

18. Brandt, *No Magic Bullet*, p. 164.

19. Hoff, *Preventive Medicine*, Vol. 5, pp. 196–198 (quotation on p. 197).

20. Treadwell, *Women's Army Corps*, pp. 615–620 (quotations on p. 616); Judith A. Bellafaire, *The Women's Army Corps: A Commemoration of World War II Service* (Washington, DC: Center of Military History, 1972); Jane Mersky Leder, *Thanks for the Memories: Love, Sex, and World War II* (Westport, CT: Praeger, 2006), pp. 44–45.

21. Ulysses Lee, *The Employment of Negro Troops* (Washington, DC: Center of Military History, 1966), pp. 71–87.

22. "United States Naval Administration in World War II," Vol. 84, "The Negro in the Navy in World War II," unpublished manuscript, Rare Book Room, Navy Department Library, http://www.ibiblio.org/hyperwar/USN/Admin-Hist/084-Negro/index.html, pp. 1–14 (quotations on p. 4).

23. Hoff, *Preventive Medicine*, Vol. 5, pp. 189–190 (quotations on p. 190).

24. "Negro in the Navy," pp. 73–74; William L. Fleming, "The Venereal Disease Problem in the United States in World War II," in *Studies in Science*, eds. William Coker and Alma Beers (Chapel Hill, NC: University of North Carolina Press, 1946), pp. 195–200; Hoff, *Preventive Medicine*, Vol. 5, p. 188.

25. Eberwein, *Sex Ed*, pp. 73–75.

26. Sue Sun Yom, "Sex and the American Soldier: Military Cinema and the War on Venereal Disease, 1918–1969," Ph.D. dissertation, University of Pennsylvania, 2003, pp. 81–82.

27. Ibid., pp. 115–116 (quotation on p. 116).

28. Hoff, *Preventive Medicine*, Vol. 5, pp. 143–146; Brandt, *No Magic Bullet*, pp. 168–169.

29. Brandt, *No Magic Bullet*, p. 170.

30. Theodore Blank, "An Historical Survey of the Development of the Use of Audio-Visual Materials in Venereal Disease Educational Programs, 1900–1949," D. Ed. dissertation, Boston University, 1970, pp. 651–664; E. Douglas Doak, "The Venereal Disease Education Institute," *Journal of Social Hygiene* 30 (1944): 12–19.

31. For examples of these posters, see Brandt, *No Magic Bullet*, between pp. 164 and 165 and Friedman, "Venereal Disease Propaganda."

32. John Parascandola, "Syphilis at the Cinema: Medicine and Morals in VD Films of the U.S. Public Health Service in World War II," in *Medicine's Moving Pictures: Medicine, Health, and Bodies in American Film and Television*, eds. Leslie J. Reagan, Nancy Tomes, and Paula A. Treichler (Rochester, NY: University of Rochester Press, 2007), pp. 71–92.

33. J. R. Heller, Jr. to C. L. Williams, September 18, 1944, PHS Records, GCR IX, 0425, "1944."

34. Press release, August 18, 1941, attached to letter from Gordon Mitchell to Raymond Vonderlehr, September 22, 1941, PHS Records, GCR X, 1350, "Know for Sure"; D. A. Dance to E. R. Coffey, August 20, 1942, PHS Records, GCR IX, 1350, "1942;" two-page typescript description of film, CDC Records, Acc. 63A788, "Know for Sure."

35. E. R. Coffey to Knox Miller, November 14, 1942; Howard Ennes, Jr. to L. C. Stoumen, May 27, 1942; E. R. Coffey to Raymond Vonderlehr, December 23, 1941, PHS Records, GCR IX, 1350, "1942."

36. Raymond Vonderlehr to Walter Clarke, February 28, 1942, PHS Records, GCR IX, 1350, "VD Film."

37. W. F. Cogswell to E. R. Coffey, April 4, 1942; E. R. Coffey to W. F. Cogswell, April 10, 1942; Raymond Vonderlehr to John Stokes, March 24, 1942; George Parkhurst to John Ankeny, February 24, 1944, PHS Records, GCR X, 1350, "Know for Sure;" Blank, "Historical Survey," p. 793.

38. Parascandola, "Syphilis at the Cinema," pp. 81–85. For another example of PHS collaboration with Hollywood on a venereal disease film, see Susan E. Lederer and John Parascandola, "Screening Syphilis: *Dr. Ehrlich's Magic Bullet* Meets the Public Health Service," *Journal of the History of Medicine* 53 (1998): 345–370.

39. "To the People of the United States" script, CDC Records, Acc. 63A788, "To the People of the United States."

40. Thomas Parran to Wilton Halverson, December 6, 1943, PHS Records, GCR IX, 1350, "1943;" Stanton Griffis to Francis Harmon, January 5, 1944; telegram from Stanton Griifis to Leroy Burney, January 6, 1944, CDC Records, Acc. 63A788, "To the People of the United States."

41. Otis Anderson to Mary Switzer, April 3, 1944, PHS Records, GCR IX, 1350, "VD Film"; Frank Walsh, *Sin and Censorship: The Catholic Church and the Motion Picture Industry* (New Haven, CT: Yale University Press, 1996), p. 180.

42. Thomas Parran to Walter Wanger, March 16, 1944, CDC Records, Acc. 63A788, "To the People of the United States."

43. "To the People of the United States" script (quotation); Walsh, *Sin and Censorship*, pp. 179–182; Thomas Parran to Wilton Halvarson, April 11, 1944, CDC Records, Acc. 63A788, "To the People of the United States."

44. "Catholics vs. V.D. Frankness," *Newsweek*, September 18, 1944, pp. 84–86 (quotations); "Catholics and Venereal Disease," *The New Republic* 111, October 9, 1944, p. 446; "Shameful, Sinful," *Time* 44, October 16, 1944: 56–57.

45. "Venereal Disease Control," prepared by United States Public Health Service and Office of War Information," January 1944, ASHA Records, box 117, folder 5.

46. *A Message to Women* (Washington, DC: Public Health Service, 1946), brochure, CDC Records, Acc. 63A314, "My Story Magazine;" *Report of the Surgeon General of the United States Public Health Service for the Fiscal Year 1946* (Washington, DC: Government Printing Office, 1946), p. 263; Eberwein, *Sex Ed*, pp. 94–95 (quotation on p. 95).

47. Examples of such posters may be found in the "Images from the History of Medicine" database of the National Library of Medicine, http://wwwihm.nlm.nih.gov. See also Brandt, *No Magic Bullet*, between pp. 164–165.

48. Brandt, *No Magic Bullet*, pp. 165–166.

49. "Relationship of the Social Protection Program to the Venereal Disease Control Program of the U.S. Public Health Service," May 20, 1942, 3-page typescript, attached to memo from L. R. Thompson to Charles P. Taft, June 17, 1942, PHS Records, GCR IX, 0425, "1942."

50. Thomas Parran to O. C. Wenger, March 23, 1942, Parran Papers, box 5, folder 38.

51. On Ness, see Paul W. Heimel, *Eliot Ness: The Real Story* (Coudersport, PA: Knox Books, 1997).

52. Ibid., p. 171.

53. "Text of Statements Presented at a National Conference on Wartime Problems in Venereal Disease Control: November 22 and 23, 1943—New York City," 10-page typescript, ASHA Records, box 117, folder 5.

54. Brandt, *No Magic Bullet*, p. 167 (quotation).

55. Ibid., p. 168.

56. "Venereal Disease Control: RTC Program," typed notes, Pritchard Papers, box 3; William G. Hollister, "The Rapid Treatment Center: A New Weapon in Venereal Disease Control," *Mississippi Doctor* 21 (1944): 316–319; Donna Pearce, "Rapid Treatment Centers for Venereal Disease Control," *American Journal of Nursing* 43 (1943): 658–660; Brandt, *No Magic Bullet*, p. 167.

57. Pearce, "Rapid Treatment," p. 658.

58. Thomas Parran to Warren G. Magnuson, March 3, 1943, PHS Records, GCR IX, 0425, box 531,"1943" (quotation); R. A. Vonderlehr to Lawrence Kolb, October 2, 1942, PHS Records, GCR IX, 0425, box 531, "1942."

59. Otis L. Anderson to R. C. Williams, July 31, 1942, PHS Records, GCR II, District 1, 0425, box 152.

60. Vonderlehr to Kolb, October 2, 1942; Ralph Chester Williams, *The United States Public Health Service, 1798–1950* (Washington, DC: Commissioned Officers Association of the United States Public Health Service, 1951), pp. 643–646.

61. *Venereal Disease Information* 24 (1943): 386; R. A. Vonderlehr to K. E. Miller, October 15, 1942, PHS Records, GCR II, District 8, 0425, box 179; Parran to Magnuson, March 3, 1943; Otis L. Anderson to A. B. Price, August 1, 1942, PHS Records, GCR II, District 4, 0425, box 168.

62. Vonderlehr to Miller, October 15, 1942; Pearce, "Rapid Treatment," p. 658; R. A. Vonderlehr to R. C. Williams, October 30, 1942, PHS Records, GCR II, District 1, 0425, box 152; "U. S. Public Health Service Outlines Policies and Responsibilities toward Rapid Treatment Centers," *Journal of Social Hygiene* 29 (1943): 239–240; Hegarty, *Victory Girls*, pp. 76–78.

63. Pearce, "Rapid Treatment"; "U.S. Public Health Service Outlines Policies"; "Rapid Treatment Centers: A Guide Designed for Use in Connection with Lanham Act Projects and Other Locally Operated Centers," January 29, 1943, Pritchard Papers, box 3.

64. J. D. Ratcliff, "The War against Syphilis," *Collier's Magazine* 111, April 10, 1943, 14–15, 72 (quotations on p. 14); Hegarty, *Victory Girls*, p. 71. On Typhoid Mary, see Judith Walzer Leavitt, *Typhoid Mary: Captive to the Public's Health* (Boston, MA: Beacon Press, 1996).

65. Ratcliff, "War against Syphilis," pp. 15, 72.

66. Hegarty, *Victory Girls*, pp. 138–141.

67. Ratcliff, "War against Syphilis," p. 72.

68. Ibid., p. 15.

69. Hollister, "The Rapid Treatment Center," p. 316.

70. Richard A. Koch and Ray Lyman Wilbur, "Promiscuity as a Factor in the Spread of Venereal Disease," *Journal of Social Hygiene* 30 (1944): 517–529 (quotations on pp. 518–519).

71. H. L. Rachlin, "A Sociologic Analysis of 304 Female Patients Admitted to the Midwestern Medical Center, St. Louis, Mo.," *Venereal Disease Information* 24 (1943): 265–271 (quotation on p. 270).

72. Ibid.; Mary Louise Webb, "Delinquency in the Making: Patterns in the Development of Girl Sex Delinquency in the City of Seattle with Recommendations for a Community Preventive Program," *Journal of Social Hygiene* 29 (1943): 502–510; James B. Hamlin, *Counseling in Rapid Treatment Centers in Relation to the Community and to the Patient* (Bethesda, MD: United States Public Health Service, 1944), copy at National Library of Medicine.

73. "Rapid Treatment Centers: A Guide," p. 3.

74. "Annual Report, U.S. Public Health Service, District No. 3, Fiscal Year 1943," 20-page typescript, PHS Records, GCR II, District 3, 1850, box 165; Hollister, "The Rapid Treatment Center," pp. 317–318; Melford S. Dickerson, "The Rapid Treatment Center Program of Texas," *Venereal Disease Information* 24 (1943): 263–265.

75. Hymen L. Rachlin to R. A. Vonderlehr, April 19, 1943, PHS Records, GCR IX, 0425, "1943;" Parran to Magnuson, March 3, 1943; "Rapid Treatment Centers: A Guide," p. 7; Florence M. Long, "Lebanon County Looks After Its Girls: A Pennsylvania Community Combats Delinquency and VD," *Journal of Social Hygiene* 31 (1945): 284–289; Francis J. Weber to W. T. Harrison, October 18, 1944, PHS Records, GCR II, District 5, 1850, box 172; "New Treatments Increase Rapid Treatment Centrer Capacity," *Journal of Social Hygiene* 31 (1945): 239–240.

76. "Rapid Treatment Centers: A Guide," p. 5; Rachlin to Vonderlehr, April 19, 1943; Hamlin, *Counseling in Rapid Treatment Centers*, p. 3.

77. "Rapid Treatment Centers: A Guide," p. 8.

78. Long, "Lebanon County," p. 287.

79. David C. Elliott to C. L. Williams, "United States Public Health Service Field Trip Report," July 3, 1943; F. M. Williams to W. E. Sowder, June 20, 1943, PHS Records, GCR II, District 3, 1850, box 169.

80. Carl C. Kuehn, "Administrative Problems in Rapid Treatment Center Operation," M. P. H. term report (thesis equivalent), University of Michigan, 1947, copy at University of Michigan Library.

81. Hegarty, *Victory Girls*, pp. 81–84 (quotation on p. 83).

82. *Venereal Disease Rapid Treatment Center*, motion picture, presented by United States Public Health Service, filmed by United States Department of Agriculture, 1944, copy at National Library of Medicine.

83. R. A. Vonderlehr to W. C. Williams, June 26, 1943; R. A. Vonderlehr to Thomas Parran, June 11, 1943; R. A. Vonderlehr to Doctor Draper, December 18, 1942, PHS Records, GCR IX, 0425, "1943" and "1942"; Charles F. Blankenship to W. T. Harrison, March 13, 1944, PHS Records, GCR II, District 5, 1850, box 172.

84. Evelyn Sarris, "A Study of 146 Patients Admitted to a Rapid Treatment Center," project submitted to National Catholic School of Social Service in partial fulfillment of requirement for Diploma in Social Work, May 1944, Washington, DC, copy at Catholic University Library; Thomas Parran, "The New War Against Venereal Disease," reprint from *Look Magazine*, 1944, Surgeons General and Other Health Administrators Speeches Collection, 1926–1963, MS C 244, National Library of Medicine, Bethesda, MD.

85. The literature on the history of penicillin is extensive. See, e.g., Robert Bud, *Penicillin: Triumph and Tragedy* (Oxford: Oxford University Press, 2007); Gladys Hobby, *Penicillin: Meeting the Challenge* (New Haven, CT: Yale University Press, 1985); Kevin Brown, *Penicillin Man: Alexander Fleming and the Antibiotic Revolution* (Stroud, UK: Sutton, 2004).

86. John Parascandola, "John Mahoney and the Introduction of Penicillin to Treat Syphilis," *Pharmacy in History* 43 (2001): 3–13; Hobby, *Penicillin*, p. 152.

87. J. F. Mahoney, R. C. Arnold, and Ad Harris, "Penicillin Treatment of Early Syphilis: A Preliminary Report," *American Journal of Public Health* 33 (1943): 1387-1391.

88. Ibid.; Hobby, *Penicillin*, pp. 155–156.

89. "New Magic Bullet," *Time* 42, October 25, 1943, pp. 38, 40.

90. J. R. Heller, Jr., "Syphilis Control in Wartime," *Southern Medical Journal* 37 (1944): 219–223 (quotation on p. 222).

91. A. N. Richards, "Production of Penicillin in the United States (1941–1946)," *Nature* 201 (1964): 441–445; J. E. Moore, "Preliminary Statement," in National Research Council—U.S. Public Health Service, *Meeting of Penicillin Investigators*, February 7 and 8 1946, p. 1 (copy at National Library of Medicine); J. F. Mahoney, R. C. Arnold, Burton L. Sterner, Ad Harris, and M. R. Zwally, "Penicillin Treatment of Early Syphilis: II," *Journal of the American Medical Association* 126 (1944): 63–67; Joseph Earle Moore, J. F. Mahoney, Walter Schwartz, Thomas Sternberg, and W. Barry Wood, "The Treatment of Early Syphilis with Penicillin: A Preliminary Report of 1,418 Cases," *Journal of the American Medical Association* 126 (1944): 67–72.

92. Richards, "Production of Penicillin," p. 444; Anderson, *Syphilis and Society*, pp. 20–21; R. A. Vonderlehr and J. R. Heller, Jr., *The Control of Venereal Disease* (New York: Reynal and Hitchcock, 1946), p. 3.

93. Henry K. Beecher, "Scarce Resources and Medical Advancement," *Daedalus* 98 (1969): 275–313 (quotation on pp. 280–81).

94. McGinnis, "From Salvarsan to Penicillin," pp. 145–146; Judith Torregrosa, "A Study of Forty-Four Syphilitic Patients Under Treatment at the Louisville Rapid Treatment Center from March 1, 1947 to April 15, 1947," M.S. in Social Work dissertation, University of Louisville, 1947 (quotation on p. v); Koch and Wilbur, "Promiscuity as a Factor"; Vonderlehr and Heller, *Control of Venereal Disease*, p. 65; Fee, "Sin vs. Science"; Brandt, *No Magic Bullet*, p. 46.

CHAPTER SIX

1. "End of Syphilis Seen by Use of Penicillin," *New York Times*, May 26, 1944; "VD Balance Sheet," *Time*, September 30, 1946; "End of Syphilis by Mass Use of Penicillin Seen," *Chicago Tribune*, February 7, 1946, p. 14.

2. R. A. Vonderlehr and J. R. Heller, Jr., *The Control of Venereal Disease* (New York: Reynal and Hitchcock, 1946), p. 64; "More Study Urged to Curb Syphilis," *The New York Times*, December 15, 1945; Evan W. Thomas, "The Function of Rapid Treatment Centers," *Journal of Social Hygiene* 33 (1947): 432–436.

3. D. O. Cauldwell, *The Latest So-Called Miracle Cure for Syphilis. Will Penicillin Go the Way of Other Cures? History and Facts about Syphilis, Its Complications and Treatment* (Girard, KS: Haldeman-Julius Publications, 1947), pp. 22–24.

4. Vonderlehr and Heller, *Control of Venereal Disease*, p. 65; Walter Clarke, "Postwar Social Hygiene Problems and Strategy," *Journal of Social Hygiene* 31 (1945): 4–15; "The New Attack on Venereal Disease," *Science Illustrated*, January 1949, pp. 29–30, 99 (quotation on p. 99).

5. Clarke, "Postwar Social Hygiene" (quotation on p. 5).

6. "Control of VD Now Urged by M'Intire," *New York Times*, October 9, 1946; "GI's Venereal Rate Sets Record Mark," *New York Times*, July 13, 1946; John Willoughby, "The Sexual Behavior of American GIs during the Early Years of the Occupation of Germany," *Journal of Military History* 62 (1998): 155–174; James R. Miller, "They Track Down VD," *Los Angeles Times*, January 5, 1947; *Social Protection*, Hearing before a Subcommittee of the Committee on Education and Labor, United States Senate, March 9, 1946 (Washington, DC: Government Printing Office, 1946), p. 1; Allan M. Brandt, *No Magic Bullet: A Social History of Venereal Disease in the United States Since 1880*, expanded edition (Oxford: Oxford University Press, 1987), appendix.

7. "The Decline of Syphilis," *Time*, February 14, 1949; "Social Disease Rate Declines in California," *Los Angeles Times*, December 20, 1950, p. 23; "VD Cases Declined in D.C. Last Year," *Washington Post*, April 19, 1951, p. 4; "Decrease in V.D. Closes One Clinic," *New York Times*, April 1, 1951, p. 76.

8. T. Green, M.D. Talbot, and R.S. Morton, "The Control of Syphilis, a Contemporary Problem: A Historical Perspective," *Sexually Transmitted Infections* 77 (2001): 214–217; Harry F. Dowling, *Fighting Infection: Conquests of the Twentieth Century* (Cambridge, MA: Harvard University Press, 1977), p. 148; "Social Hygienists Say War against Venereal Disease Is Almost Won," *Washington Post*, May 20, 1953, p. 25; Elizabeth W. Etheridge, *Sentinel for Health: A History of the Centers for Disease Control* (Berkeley, CA: University of California Press, 1992), p. 90.

9. "End of Syphilis in Sight, Says Medical Expert," *Chicago Daily Tribune*, December 7, 1950, p. A10; John F. Mahoney, "The Effects of the Antibiotics on the Concepts and Practices of Public Health," in *The Impact of the Antibiotics on Medicine and Society*, ed. Iago Galdston (New York: International Universities Press, 1958), pp. 207–217 (quotation on p. 210).

10. "Warning is Given on Venereal Ills," *New York Times*, March 7, 1953, p. 21; "Hidden Cases of VD Listed as 2 Million," *Washington Post*, May 14, 1953, p. 10; "Slight Rise in Venereal Cases Noted," *Washington Post*, January 31, 1954, p. C7; "VD Rate Rises in 25 States," *Washington Post*, February 1, 1956, p. 20; "Cases of Syphilis Increase in Year," *New York Times*, February 14, 1947, p. 24.

11. "Venereal Cases Declared Rising," *New York Times*, November 10, 1959, p. 35; Etheridge, *Sentinel for Health*, pp. 87–92.

12. Odin W. Anderson, *Syphilis and Society—Problems of Control in the United States, 1912–1964* (Chicago: Center for Health Administration Studies, Health Information Foundation,

1965), pp. 22–33, 53; "VD Survey Sought," *New York Times*, February 23, 1954, p. 21; Brandt, *No Magic Bullet*, pp. 174–178.

13. William J. Brown, "Let's Stamp Out VD Now!" *Los Angeles Times*, September 18, 1960, p. TW20; "Teen-Age VD," *Time*, April 7, 1961; Brandt, *No Magic Bullet*, p. 174.

14. Brown, "Stamp Out VD."

15. Brandt, *No Magic Bullet*, p. 175.

16. Brandt, *No Magic Bullet*, pp. 176–178.

17. Ibid., p. 176; "The Way to Sex Education," *New York Times*, June 2, 1969; "Storm Over the Teaching of Sex," *New York Times*, September 7, 1969; "Surgeon General Pleads for Story," *New York Times*, November 17, 1964; "VD Posters Covered for Lunch Guests," *Washington Post*, June 1, 1956, p. 33.

18. Ira L. Schamberg, "Syphilis and Sisyphus," *British Journal of Venereal Disease* 39 (1963): 87–97; Crawford F. Sams, *"Medic:" The Mission of an American Military Doctor in Occupied Japan and Wartorn Korea* (Armonk, NY: M. E. Sharpe, 1998), p. 107.

19. Anderson, *Syphilis and Society*, pp. 38–39; Public Health Service, *The Eradication of Syphilis: A Task Force Report to the Surgeon General Public Health Service on Syphilis Control in the United States* (Washington, DC: Government Printing Office, 1962), p. ii; Leona Baumgartner, "Syphilis Eradication—A Plan for Action Now," in *Proceedings of World Forum on Syphilis and Other Treponematoses, Washington, D.C., September 4–8, 1962* (Washington, DC: Government Printing Office, 1964), pp. 26–32.

20. Leona Baumgartner to Luther Terry, December 29, 1961, in Public Health Service, *Eradication of Syphilis*, p. 2.

21. Public Health Service, *Eradication of Syphilis*, pp. 29–30.

22. Untitled typescript of talk delivered by William Brown at Venereal Disease Conference, University of Oklahoma, November 6, 1965, CDC Records, Acc. 70A470, VD Manuscript Files, 1965–1966. See also William Brown, "Progress of the Syphilis Eradication Program in the United States," typescript of talk given at United States–Mexico Border Meeting, Los Angeles, June 7–10, 1965, CDC Records, Acc. 71A1708, VD Manuscript Files, 1964–1966, 1967–1968.

23. Public Health Advisory Committee on Venereal Disease Control, *A Follow-up Report of the Surgeon General's Task Force on Syphilis Control* (Atlanta, GA: National Communicable Disease Center, 1966), pp. iv, 1–4, copy in CDC Records, Acc. 68A1665, VD Programs, 1961–1968.

24. "Report of the Venereal Disease Program Fiscal Year 1967," CDC Records, Acc. 71A708, Manuscript Files, 1964–1966, 1967–1968; Brandt, *No Magic Bullet*, Appendix.

25. "U.S. Panel Urges a Drive to Control V.D.," *New York Times*, April 5, 1972, p. 1.

26. Mark R. Grandstaff, "Making the Military American: Advertising, Reform, and the Demise of an Antistanding Military Tradition, 1945–1955," *Journal of Military History* 60 (1996): 299–324 (quotation on p. 318).

27. Ibid., pp. 319–321.

28. Albert E. Cowdrey, *The Medics' War* (Washington, DC: Center of Military History, United States Army, 1987), pp. 148–149, 183–184 (quotation from Pierce is on p. 184).

29. Ibid., p. 249.

30. Katharine H. S. Moon, *Sex among Allies: Military Prostitution in U.S.–Korea Relations* (New York: Columbia University Press, 1997).

31. Sue Sun Yom, "Sex and the American Soldier: Military Cinema and the War on Venereal Disease, 1918–1969," Ph.D. dissertation, University of Pennsylvania, 2003, pp. 126–136 (quotations on p. 126–127); James F. Dunnigan and Albert A. Nofi, *Dirty Little Secrets of the Vietnam War* (New York: St. Martin's Griffin: 2000), pp. 165–166; Kathleen Barry, *The Prostitution of Sexuality* (New York: New York University Press, 1995), p. 132.

32. Susan Brownmiller, *Against Our Will: Men, Women and Rape* (New York: Fawcett Columbine, 1975), pp. 93–95; Barry, *Prostitution*, pp. 130–135.

33. James E. Westheider, *Fighting on Two Fronts: African Americans and the Vietnam War* (New York: New York University Press, 1997), p. 117; Brownmiller, *Against Our Will*, pp. 96–97.

34. Yom, "Sex and the American Soldier," pp. 127–130 (quotation on pp. 129–130).

35. Brownmiller, *Against Our Will*, p. 96; Dunnigan and Nofi, *Dirty Little Secrets*, p. 166; Paul C. White and Joseph H. Blount, "Venereal Disease Control in the 2nd Marine Division, Camp Lejeune, North Carolina," *Military Medicine* 132 (1967): 252–257; S. R. Shapiro and L. C. Breschi, "Venereal Disease in Vietnam: Clinical Experience at a Major Military Hospital," *Military Medicine* 139 (1974): 374–379.

36. Monte Gulzow and Carol Mitchell, "'Vagina Denta' and 'Incurable Venereal Disease' Legends from the Viet Nam War," *Western Folklore* 39 (1980): 306–316; Herb Friedman, "Venereal Disease Propaganda," http://www.psywarrior.com/PSYOPVD.html.

37. Etheridge, *Sentinel for Health*, pp. 235–237.

38. "Venereal Disease Cases Up," *The Post* (Frederick, MD), March 3, 1975, p. A3; "Venereal Disease Slowing," *Warren Times Observer* (Warren, OH), March 16, 1977, p. 11; Brandt, *No Magic Bullet*, appendix.

39. On the history of AIDS, see Brandt, *No Magic Bullet*, pp. 183–204; Mirko D. Grmek, *History of AIDS: Emergence and Origin of a Modern Pandemic*, trans. by Russell C. Maulitz and Jacalyn Duffin (Princeton, NJ: Princeton University Press, 1990); Elizabeth Fee and Daniel M. Fox, *AIDS: The Burdens of History* (Berkeley, CA: University of California Press, 1988); Caroline Hannaway, Victoria A. Harden, and John Parascandola, eds., *AIDS and the Public Debate* (Amsterdam: IOS Press, 1995).

40. William Benemann, *Male-Male Intimacy in Early America: Beyond Romantic Friendships* (Binghamton, NY: Haworth Press, 2006), pp. 135–138.

41. One early article of this period on the subject reflects the contemporary attitudes toward homosexuality in its title. See H. Goodman, "An Epidemic of Genital Chancres from Perversion," *American Journal of Syphilis, Gonorrhea, and Venereal Disease* 28 (1944): 310–314.

42. Bernard F. Rosenblum, "Homosexuality in Venereal Disease," typescript of talk intended for presentation to Western Branch American Public Health Association and United States-Mexico Border Public Health Association,1961, attached to letter from William J. Brown to Rosenblum, June 7, 1961; Maxim Demchak, "The Problem of the Homosexual in Venereal Disease Control," typescript of talk presented to the Venereal Disease Committee of the North Caroline State Medical Society, September 27, 1963, attached to letter from William J. Brown to Demchak, November 14, 1963, CDC Records, Acc. 70A470, Manuscript Files, 1961–1966; Annet Mooij, *Out of Otherness: Characters and Narrators in the Dutch Venereal Disease Debates 1850–1990* (Amsterdam: Editions Rodopi, 1998), pp. 180–188.

43. Rosenblum, "Homosexuality;" Demchak, "The Problem of the Homosexual."

44. Centers for Disease Control and Prevention, *Sexually Transmitted Disease Surveillance 2003 Supplement, Syphilis Surveillance Report* (Atlanta, GA: Centers for Disease Control and Prevention, 2004), pp. 25–28.

45. Centers for Disease Control and Prevention, *The National Plan to Eliminate Syphilis from the United States* (Atlanta, GA: Centers for Disease Control and Prevention, 1999), pp. 5–6.

46. "Overall Syphilis Rate Rises for First Time Since 1990," press release, Centers for Disease Control and Prevention, November 1, 2002, http://www.cdc.gov/od/oc/media/pressrel/r021101b.htm; Timothy F. Kirn, "Syphilis Rates Continue 5-Year Rise, Driven by Male-to-Male Sex," *Internal Medicine News* 38 (December 1, 2005): 7.

47. N. C. Grassly, C. Fraser, and G. P. Garnett, "Host Immunity and Synchronized Epidemics of Syphilis across the United States," *Nature* 433 (2007): 417–421; "Syphilis Rates Cyclical?" *CBS News*, January 26, 2005, http://www.cbsnews.com/stories/2005/01/26/health/main669589.shtml.

48. Paul A. Cullen and Caroline E. Cameron, "Progress towards an Effective Syphilis Vaccine: The Past, Present and Future," *Expert Review of Vaccines* 5 (2006): 67–80.

49. Walter Sullivan, "Venereal Disease," *New York Times*, May 5, 1964; "Syphilis Vaccine Gains," *New York Times*, December 9, 1954, p. 26; Nate Haseltine, "Syphilis Preventive Suggested Possible," *Washington Post and Times Herald*, October 17, 1954, p. B2; George Getze, "Syphilis Vaccine May Result from UCLA Work," *Los Angeles Times*, June 30, 1967, p. A6; S. A. Lukehart, "Progress toward Development of a Vaccine for Syphilis," *Abstracts of the Interscience Conference on Antimicrobial Agents, and Chemotherapy* 40 (2000): 540; Ellen Licking, "Inching Closer to a Syphilis Vaccine," *Business Week Online*, September 20, 2000, http://www.businessweek.com/bwdaily/dnflash/sep2000/nf20000920_834.htm; Richard D. Lyons, "New Study Seeks Syphilis Vaccine," *New York Times*, June 21, 1968, p. 16; Lawrence K. Altman, "Polish Research Team Reports Early Successes in Testing Experimental Syphilis Vaccine in Rabbits," *New York Times*, June 9, 1971, p. 21; Lawrence K. Altman, "Syphilis Vaccine is Tested after Bacterium is Grown," *New York Times*, March 13, 1976, p. 1.

50. Lukehart, "Progress"; Licking, "Inching Closer."

51. See, e.g., Rebecca E. LaFond and Sheila A. Lukehart, "Biological Basis for Syphilis," *Clinical Microbiology Reviews* 19 (2006): 29–49.

52. Harrell W. Chesson, Steven D. Pinkerton, Richard Voigt, and George W. Counts, "HIV Infections and Associated Costs Attributable to Syphilis Coinfection among African Americans," *American Journal of Public Health* 93 (2003): 943–948; Michael E. Blocker, William C. Levine, and Michael E. St. Louis, "HIV Prevalence in Patients with Syphilis, United States," *Sexually Transmitted Diseases* 27 (2000): 53–59; J. R. Berger, M. McCarthy, L. Resnick, M. A. Fletcher, N. Klimas, and L. La Voie, "History of Syphilis as a Cofactor for the Expression of HIV Infection," *V International Conference on AIDS*, June 4–9, 1989, p. 93; John Crewdson, "Weak Immune System May Open AIDS Door," *Chicago Tribune*, December 20, 1987, p. 1.

53. Centers for Disease Control and Prevention, *Report of the Syphilis Elimination Efforts Consultation, August 1–2, 2005* (Atlanta, GA: Centers for Disease Control and Prevention, 2005); Centers for Disease Control and Prevention, *The National Plan to Eliminate Syphilis from the United States* (Atlanta, GA: Centers for Disease Control and Prevention, 2006) (quotation on p. vii).

54. Brandt, *No Magic Bullet*, pp. 183–204 (quotation on p. 199); Allan M. Brandt, "The Syphilis Epidemic and Its Relation to AIDS," *Science* 239 (1988): 375–380; Allan M. Brandt, "AIDS in Historical Perspective: Four Lessons from the History of Sexually Transmitted Diseases," *American Journal of Public Health* 78 (1988): 367–371.

55. Perry Treadwell, *God's Judgment? Syphilis and AIDS* (San Jose, CA: Writers Club Press, 2001) (quotation on p. xi).

56. C. Everett Koop, *Koop: The Memoirs of America's Family Doctor* (New York: Random House, 1991), pp. 194–239; United States Public Health Service, Office of the Surgeon General, *Surgeon General's Report on Acquired Immune Deficiency Syndrome* (United States Public Health Service, Office of the Surgeon General, 1986); United States Public Health Service, Office of the Surgeon General and Centers for Disease Control, *Understanding AIDS* (U.S. Department of Health and Human Services, 1988).

57. Treadwell, *God's Judgment*, pp. 48–50; Brandt, *No Magic Bullet*, pp. 188–199; Koop, *Memoirs*, pp. 227–230; "Poll Indicates Majority Favors Quarantine for AIDS Victims," *New York Times*, December 20, 1985.

58. Brandt, "AIDS in Historical Perspective."

59. Rosemary A. Stevens, "Health Care in the Early 1960s," *Health Care Financing Review* 18 (1996): 11–22; Joshua Lederberg, "Infectious History," *Science* 288 (2000): 287–293; Institute of Medicine, *Emerging Infections: Microbial Threats to Health in the United States* (Washington, DC: National Academy Press, 1992).

60. Brandt, *No Magic Bullet*, p. 199.

BIBLIOGRAPHY

I have drawn upon a large number and wide variety of primary and secondary sources in the preparation of this book, as reflected in the chapter notes. The literature on the history of venereal disease, prostitution, sexuality, and related topics is extensive. I have listed below those works that I found most useful for my purposes. This bibliography should also be helpful to the reader who wishes to explore the subject further.

ARCHIVES AND MANUSCRIPTS

I have consulted the following archival collections in my research. In the chapter notes, the references to these collections have been abbreviated as shown in parentheses following the entries below.

American Social Hygiene Association Records, Social Welfare History Archives, Elmer L. Andersen Library, University of Minnesota, Minneapolis, MN (ASHA Records).

Centers for Disease Control and Prevention Records, Record Group 442, National Archives and Records Administration, Southeast Region, Morrow, GA (CDC Records).

Records of the Council on National Defense, 1915–1937, Record Group 62, Committee for Civilian Cooperation in Combating Venereal Diseases Records, 1917–1918, National Archives and Records Administration, College Park, MD (CCCCVD Records).

Papers of Thomas Parran, 1916–1962, Record Group 90/F14, Archives Service Center, University of Pittsburgh, Pittsburgh, PA (Parran Papers).

Elizabeth Gatlin Pritchard Papers, 1902–1963, MS C 187, History of Medicine Division, National Library of Medicine, Bethesda, MD (Pritchard Papers).

Public Health Service Records, Record Group 90, General Classified Records, 1936–1944, National Archives and Records Administration, College Park, MD (PHS Records GCR).

Public Health Service Records, Record Group 90, Records of the Division of Venereal Diseases, National Archives and Records Administration, College Park, MD (PHS DVD Records).

Records of the War Department General and Special Staffs, Record Group 165, Commission on Training Camp Activities Records, National Archives and Records Administration, College Park, MD (CTCA Records).

BOOKS

Alexander, Ruth M. *The "Girl Problem": Female Sexual Delinquency in New York, 1900–1930* (Ithaca, NY: Cornell University Press, 1995).

Allen, Peter Lewis. *The Wages of Sin: Sex and Disease, Past and Present* (Chicago: University of Chicago Press, 2000).

Anderson, Odin W. *Syphilis and Society—Problems of Control in the United States, 1912–1964* (Chicago: Center for Health Administration Studies, Health Information Foundation, 1965).

Arrizabalaga, Jon, John Henderson, and Roger French. *The Great Pox: The French Disease in Renaissance Europe* (New Haven, CT: Yale University Press, 1997).

Brandt, Allan M. *No Magic Bullet: A Social History of Venereal Disease in the United States Since 1880*, expanded edition (Oxford: Oxford University Press, 1987).

Bristow, Nancy R. *Making Men Moral: Social Engineering during the Great War* (New York: New York University Press, 1996).

Bullough, Vern L. *The History of Prostitution* (New Hyde Park, NY: University Books, 1964).

Cassel, Jay. *The Secret Plague: Venereal Disease in Canada 1838–1939* (Toronto: University of Toronto Press, 1987).

Centers for Disease Control and Prevention. *The National Plan to Eliminate Syphilis from the United States* (Atlanta, GA: Centers for Disease Control and Prevention, 1999).

———. *Report of the Syphilis Elimination Efforts Consultation, August 1–2, 2005* (Atlanta, GA: Centers for Disease Control and Prevention, 2005).

———. *The National Plan to Eliminate Syphilis from the United States* (Atlanta, GA: Centers for Disease Control and Prevention, 2006).

Davidson, Roger. *Dangerous Liaisons: A Social History of Venereal Disease in Twentieth-Century Scotland* (Amsterdam: Editions Rodopi, 2000).

Davidson, Roger and Lesley A. Hall, eds. *Sex, Sin and Suffering: Venereal Disease and European Society since 1870* (London: Routledge, 2001).

D'Emilio, John and Estelle B. Freedman. *Intimate Matters: A History of Sexuality in America*, 2nd ed. (Chicago: University of Chicago Press, 1997).

Dietzler, Mary Marcy. *Detention Houses and Reformatories as Protective Social Agencies in the Campaign of the United States Government against Venereal Disease* (Washington, DC: Government Printing Office, 1922).

Eberwein, Robert. *Sex Ed: Film, Video, and the Framework of Desire* (New Brunswick, NJ: Rutgers University Press, 1999).

Gihon, Albert L. *Report of the Committee on the Prevention of Venereal Diseases* (Boston, MA: Franklin Press: Rand, Avery, and Company, 1881).

Godbeer, Richard. *Sexual Revolution in Early America* (Baltimore, MD: Johns Hopkins University Press, 2002).

Hayden, Deborah. *Pox: Genius, Madness, and the Mysteries of Syphilis* (New York: Basic Books, 2003).

Hegarty, Marilyn E. *Victory Girls, Khaki-Wackies, and Patriotutes: The Regulation of Female Sexuality in World War II* (New York: New York University Press, 2008).

Hobson, Barbara Meil. *Uneasy Virtue: The Politics of Prostitution and the American Reform Tradition* (New York: Basic Books, 1987).

Hoff, Ebbe Curtiss, ed. *Preventive Medicine in World War II*, nine volumes (Washington, DC: Office of the Surgeon General, Department of the Army, 1955–1969).

Jones, James H. *Bad Blood: The Tuskegee Syphilis Experiment*, new and expanded edition (New York: Free Press, 1993).

Lowry, Thomas P. *Venereal Disease and the Lewis and Clark Expedition* (Lincoln, NE: University of Nebraska Press, 2004).

Merians, Linda E., ed. *The Secret Malady: Venereal Disease in Eighteenth-Century Britain and France* (Lexington, KY: University Press of Kentucky, 1997).

Mooij, Annet. *Out of Otherness: Characters and Narrators in the Dutch Venereal Disease Debates 1850–1990* (Amsterdam: Editions Rodopi, 1998).

Odem, Mary E. *Delinquent Daughters: Protecting and Policing Adolescent Female Sexuality in the United States, 1885–1920* (Chapel Hill, NC: University of North Carolina Press, 1995).

Parran, Thomas. *Shadow on the Land: Syphilis* (New York: Reynal and Hitchcock, 1937).

Parran, Thomas and Raymond Vonderlehr. *Plain Words about Venereal Disease* (New York: Reynal and Hitchcock, 1941).

Poirier, Suzanne. *Chicago's War on Syphilis, 1937–1940: The Times, the Trib, and the Clap Doctor* (Urbana, IL: University of Illinois Press, 1995).

Powell, Mary Lucas and Della Collins Cook, eds. *The Myth of Syphilis: The Natural History of Treponematosis in North America* (Gainesville, FL: University Press of Florida, 2005).

Public Health Service. *The Eradication of Syphilis: A Task Force Report to the Surgeon General Public Health Service on Syphilis Control in the United States* (Washington, DC: Government Printing Office, 1962).

Quétel, Claude. *History of Syphilis*. Translated into English by Judith Braddock and Brian Pike (Baltimore, MD: Johns Hopkins University Press, 1990).

Reverby, Susan M., ed. *Tuskegee's Truths: Rethinking the Tuskegee Syphilis Study* (Chapel Hill, NC: University of North Caroline Press, 2000).

Rosebury, Theodor. *Microbes and Morals: The Strange Story of Venereal Disease* (New York: Viking Press, 1971).

Siena, Kevin P. *Venereal Disease, Hospitals and the Urban Poor: London's "Foul Wards," 1600–1800* (Rochester, NY: University of Rochester Press, 2004).

———, ed. *Sins of the Flesh: Responding to Sexual Disease in Early Modern Europe* (Toronto: Centre for Reformation and Renaissance Studies, 2005).

Spongberg, Mary. *Feminizing Venereal Disease: The Body of the Prostitute in Nineteenth-Century Medical Discourse* (New York: New York University Press, 1997).

Vonderlehr, R. A. and J. R. Heller, Jr. *The Control of Venereal Disease* (New York: Reynal and Hitchcock, 1946).

DISSERTATIONS

Blank, Theodore. "An Historical Survey of the Development of the Use of Audio-Visual Materials in Venereal Disease Educational Programs, 1900–1949." D. Ed. dissertation, Boston University, 1970, pp. 651–664.

Janke, Linda Sharon. "Prisoners of War: Sexuality, Venereal Disease, and Women's Incarceration during World War I." Ph.D. dissertation, Binghamton University, State University of New York, 2006.

Rockafellar, Nancy Moore. "Making the World Safe for the Soldiers of Democracy: Patriotism, Public Health and Venereal Disease Control on the West Coast, 1910–1919." Ph.D. dissertation, University of Washington, 1990.

Yom, Sue Sun. "Sex and the American Soldier: Military Cinema and the War on Venereal Disease, 1918–1969." Ph.D. dissertation, University of Pennsylvania, 2003.

ARTICLES

Note: Articles published or reprinted in the books listed earlier are not included in the following list.

Beardsley, Edward H. "Allied against Sin: American and British Responses to Venereal Disease in World War I." *Medical History* 20 (1976): 189–202.

Brandt, Allan M. "The Syphilis Epidemic and Its Relation to AIDS." *Science* 239 (1988): 375–380.

———. "AIDS in Historical Perspective: Four Lessons from the History of Sexually Transmitted Diseases." *American Journal of Public Health* 78 (1988): 367–371.

Burney, Leroy E. "Control of Syphilis in a Southern Rural Area." *American Journal of Public Health* 29 (1939): 1006–1014.

Burnham, John C. "Medical Inspection of Prostitutes in the Nineteenth Century: The St. Louis Experiment and Its Sequel." *Bulletin of the History of Medicine* 45 (1971): 203–218.

Clarke, Walter. "Postwar Social Hygiene Problems and Strategy." *Journal of Social Hygiene* 31 (1945): 4–15.

Dracobly, Alex. "Ethics and Experimentation on Human Subjects in Mid-Nineteenth-Century France: The Story of the 1859 Syphilis Experiments." *Bulletin of the History of Medicine* 77 (2003): 332–366.

Fee, Elizabeth. "Sin vs. Science: Venereal Disease in Baltimore in the Twentieth Century." *Bulletin of the History of Medicine* 43 (1988): 141–164.

Foa, Anna. "The New and the Old: The Spread of Syphilis (1494–1530)." Translated into English by Carole C. Gallucci, in *Sex and Gender in Historical Perspective*, eds. Edward Muir and Guido Ruggiero (Baltimore, MD: Johns Hopkins University Press, 1990), pp. 26–45.

Gould, Stephen Jay "Syphilis and the Shepherd of Atlantis," *Natural History* 109 (October 2000): 38–42, 74–82.

Gross, S. D. "Syphilis in Its Relation to the National Health." *Transactions of the American Medical Association* 25 (1874): 249–292.

Hollister, William G. "The Rapid Treatment Center: A New Weapon in Venereal Disease Control." *Mississippi Doctor* 21 (1944): 316–319.

Imber, Michael. "The First World War, Sex Education, and the American Social Hygiene Association's Campaign against Venereal Disease." *Journal of Educational History and Administration* 16 (1984): 47–56.

Jones, James Boyd, Jr. "A Tale of Two Cities: The Hidden Battle against Venereal Disease in Civil War Nashville and Memphis." *Civil War History* 31 (1985): 270–276.

Kampmeier, Rudolph H. "Syphilis Therapy: An Historical Perspective," *Journal of the American Venereal Disease Association* 3 (1976): 99–108.

———. "Venereal Disease in the United States Army: 1775–1900." *Sexually Transmitted Diseases* 9 (1982): 100–103.

Larimore, Granville W. and Thomas H. Sternberg. "Does Health Education Prevent Venereal Disease? The Army's Experience with 8,000,000 Men." *American Journal of Public Health* 35 (1945): 799–804.

Lederer, Susan E. and John Parascandola. "Screening Syphilis: *Dr. Ehrlich's Magic Bullet* Meets the Public Health Service," *Journal of the History of Medicine* 53 (1998): 345–370.

Long, Florence M. "Lebanon County Looks after Its Girls: A Pennsylvania Community Combats Delinquency and VD," *Journal of Social Hygiene* 31 (1945): 284–289.

Mahoney, J. F., R. C. Arnold, and Ad Harris. "Penicillin Treatment of Early Syphilis: A Preliminary Report." *American Journal of Public Health* 33 (1943): 1387–1391.

McGinnis, Janice Dickin. "From Salvarsan to Penicillin: Medical Science and VD Control in Canada," in *Essays in the History of Canadian Medicine*, eds. Wendy Mitchinson and Janice Dicken McGinnis (Toronto: McClelland and Stewart, 1988), pp. 126–147.

Meyer, C., C. Jung, T. Kohl, A. Poenicke, A. Poppe, and K. W. Alt, "Syphilis 2001—A Paleontological Reappraisal." *Homo* 53 (2002): 39–58.

Miles, Toni P. and David McBride. "World War I Origins of the Syphilis Epidemic among 20th Century Black Americans: A Biohistorical Analysis." *Social Science & Medicine* 45 (1997): 61–69.

Murphy, Lawrence R. "The Enemy among Us: Venereal Disease among Union Soldiers in the Far West, 1861–1865." *Civil War History* 31 (1985): 257–269.

Parascandola, John. "John Mahoney and the Introduction of Penicillin to Treat Syphilis." *Pharmacy in History* 43 (2001): 3–13.

———. "Syphilis at the Cinema: Medicine and Morals in VD Films of the U.S. Public Health Service in World War II," in *Medicine's Moving Pictures: Medicine, Health, and Bodies in American Film and Television*, eds. Leslie J. Reagan, Nancy Tomes, and Paula A. Treichler (Rochester, NY: University of Rochester Press, 2007), pp. 71–92.

Parran, Thomas. "Syphilis Can Be Stamped Out," *Readers Digest*, April 1937, pp. 21–25.

Pearce, Donna. "Rapid Treatment Centers for Venereal Disease Control." *American Journal of Nursing* 43 (1943): 658–660.

Ratcliff, J. D. "The War against Syphilis." *Collier's Magazine* 111 (April 10, 1943): 14–15, 72.

Sartin, Jeffrey S. and Harold O. Perry. "From Mercury to Malaria to Penicillin: The History of the Treatment of Syphilis at the Mayo Clinic—1916–1955." *Journal of the American Academy of Dermatology* 32 (1995): 255–261.

Sherwood, Joan. "Syphilization: Human Experimentation in the Search for a Syphilis Vaccine in the Nineteenth Century." *Bulletin of the History of Medicine* 54 (1999): 364–386.

"U. S. Public Health Service Outlines Policies and Responsibilities toward Rapid Treatment Centers." *Journal of Social Hygiene* 29 (1943): 239–240.

Walls, Edwina. "Hot Springs Waters and the Treatment of Venereal Diseases: The U. S. Public Health Service Clinic and Camp Garraday." *Journal of the Arkansas Medical Society* 91 (1995): 430–437.

INDEX

About the Author

JOHN PARASCANDOLA is a lecturer in the Department of History at the University of Maryland. He has served as Chief of the History of Medicine Division of the National Library of Medicine, after which he became the Public Health Service Historian, a position he held until his retirement in 1992. He is also the author of *The Development of American Pharmacology: John J. Abel and the Shaping of a Discipline* (1992).